GASTRIC SURGERY: THE LIVED EXPERIENCE

WHAT TO EXPECT PRE AND POST-SURGERY

LOUISE NEIL

DISCLAIMER

The information given in this book should not be treated as a substitute for medical advice. Always consult a medical practitioner before embarking on any weight loss plan. Any use of the information in this book is at the reader's discretion and risk. Neither the author nor the publisher can be held responsible for any loss, claim or damage arising out of the use, or misuse, of the examples given, the suggestions made, the failure to take medical advice or for any material on third-party websites.

DEDICATION

To the old Louise. You went through so much, not just with your weight. I didn't always put you first, however, I will always do my best for you and continue to improve our new life.

ACKNOWLEDGEMENTS

To my Grandad. He never commented on my weight, ever. He was always kind and graceful, he saw my potential, as he did with all of us. He was a true gentleman.

To my mum, who supported me financially when she knew my decision was made and to my dad, who makes a mean, high-protein consommé soup. Both of them looked after me post-op and for that, I am forever grateful.

To my children, who without realising, have been with me every step of the gastric surgery journey. With their love, kindness and immediate acceptance of their changing mum, I love them unconditionally.

To my brother, cousins wider family and friends, old and new. Those who have stood by me regardless of weight, decisions or situations. You have been there for me and for that I owe you a drink, cheers.

To my husband. Who accepted me for who I am from the moment we met, which was post-surgery. He is my major cheerleader. He nurtures me to ensure I can be the best version of myself. I love him deeply, he keeps me warm, cooks for me and dyes my hair pretty well too.

And finally, to my surgeon, Mr Michael Van den Bossche who has no idea I have written this book nor the long-standing and far-reaching positive impact he and his team have had on my life. You created the first step in my transformation.

CONTENTS

INTRODUCTION

My name is Louise.

I have had Gastric Surgery.

Welcome to our book, Gastric Surgery: The Lived Experience

I say our book because it is for you and me, together. To share my experience and by doing so, to support you through yours.

After more than six successful years as a Gastric Surgery patient, I have decided to write my story, sharing my journey and many of my experiences with you, so that you can benefit from them, learn from them, and so that my journey can support your future success.

By investing in this book, you will either be considering gastric surgery, have had gastric surgery, or be supporting someone you love through gastric surgery. Potentially, you may just be being nosey and want to find out what it is actually like to go through the gastric surgery process, and why not?

I am writing about my own personal journey. There is no medical advice in this book, just raw personal experiences mixed with potential solutions based on these experiences - the ones that I wish someone had shared with me prior to and post-surgery.

You won't find any medical jargon or advice from the medical professionals - you must go to them for that. This book is written with you in mind, it is personal and to the point. It includes, you know, the sort of stuff you need to know to go along with all of the medical advice, the nitty gritty stuff that no one talks about. It also covers the stuff that may seem quite simple once you have been through it but if you haven't, you may not really know where to go for the answer or may not even know that a particular experience was a "thing".

I hope to answer a lot of your questions and I also aim to make you laugh. You will be able to relate directly to many things I have been through, whether you have already been through them (and if you have, we can high five should we ever meet), or if you haven't - in which case, you can learn from them in readiness for what you may go through, should you have gastric surgery. If you are reading to support someone you know and love going through gastric surgery, then this book is going to really open your eyes to what it is like to be a gastric surgery patient.

1986 was the first time that I realised I was not as lean as my friend. I was seven years old. Well, I didn't work it out for myself as I didn't see myself as overweight, in fact, I don't think I had ever seen anyone as anything bar what they were: human, nice, friendly, and fun. I was aware there were people in life who were not nice, however until that day, I had not ever computed that I was on the overweight side of things and that people saw being overweight as an actual issue. If I thought really hard, I could probably pinpoint the date that I was shocked into reality. I had a lovely upbringing, and a nice brother, my parents both worked and they were fun and kind. We enjoyed sports and spending time together when work and school allowed. At times when our parents were doing well, we were spoiled and when they weren't, we weren't. We were your run-of-the-mill kinda family where everyone mucked in, got along, enjoyed life and made the best of things.

It was mid-week and I was at a friend's house for tea as it was her birthday. What went from being an exciting day at school as we built up to the end of the day, suddenly and completely changed my life. It changed my mindset and impacted my life in so many ways, quite literally from that moment forward. We were having a really nice time and were called to the dinner table. Out of nowhere, her mum said *"You like your food Louise, I hope I have enough!"* I can remember saying, *"It's ok, I have lots thank you"*, and her mum said, whilst laughing *"It's not quite what I meant"*. I can remember looking at my friend and could feel my cheeks burning. My friend looked embarrassed and didn't say anything, and my tummy was telling me she wasn't being nice and it felt uncomfortable. We went on to have a nice hour or so after dinner before I was picked up by my mum. No one said anything at the front door, so I never said anything to my Mum. From the following day, it was different with my friend, she wasn't really my friend any more, her mum's comments had affected our friendship and, slowly but surely, our friendship ended and other children that had been there also began to tease me, on and off, about my weight. I was a confident girl, however, I went from being confident in a relaxed manner to being nervously confident, I would describe it as almost anxious. I have never actually shared that with anyone before. No one. Whoever reads this first is the first to know this information, that 1986 was the first time I had been made to feel uncomfortable about my own body and that one incident impacted my whole future.

Looking back, it was a horrible situation to be in and certainly impacted my life's trajectory, it set my identity which impacted me for years, however, as an adult, I have learnt important lessons and choose to be grateful that it built resilience in me and I have mastered my beliefs of myself, e.g. I am a healthy weight and make good food and drink choices, which has enabled me to change my identity hand in hand with my gastric surgery. Now, I am not sure if I naturally have strong resilience, if I learned to have it, or both. Later in the book, I talk more about resilience and another topic that supports it. I am sure you will have had experiences like it, the ones that literally take away a piece of your soul each time they happen. This was another driver for me with Gastric Surgery: The Lived Experience, to give as many people who have been through similar, back a piece of their soul. I want everyone to know, those of you who have struggled with your weight for whatever reason, and for those of us who have chosen to have gastric surgery, I hear you, I stand with you, and you are not alone.

Over the course of my teenage years and early 20s, my weight fluctuated up and down and it simply depended on how I was feeling, where I was living and what I was doing.

If I had a job where I was on my feet moving around, happy and excited with life, my weight was stable and I was a relatively healthy weight. If I was studying or had a very sedentary or stressful job, my weight would increase and I would eat more, likely due to boredom and habit, however almost certainly linked to emotional responses. Interestingly, it is those times that really taught me what I could do to protect my weight loss post-surgery.

Fast forward 30 years. It is 2016 and I decided to have gastric surgery. When I had my surgery, it was still fairly unknown and an unspoken thing to do. People had gotten over the taboo subject of cosmetic surgery and would freely discuss it. People having boob jobs no longer created a shock or was a thing to talk about. In 2016, I remember botox becoming the norm and then lip fillers slowly making their way into people's faces just like botox had. However, if anyone mentioned gastric surgery, well, blimey, that was still a taboo subject and shocked most people. It still often does, although not as much as it did back in 2016.

When I decided to have surgery, I had already spoken to my GP at length. I was at the end of trying to lose weight yet again and stabilise my weight loss for the long term. I disclosed that this was also impacted due to being in an unhappy and difficult marriage and I knew I had basically become worn out, especially with having to always battle my weight and my mind and everything else that goes with it, including people's comments and reactions, conscious and unconscious. There was, and still is, an NHS referral system, a staged process, which I was put into, however, I was rejected. During this period I had mapped out a plan to change my life and I had already decided that I would seek private surgery if I didn't meet the NHS criteria. I would be having it done anyway, by hook or by crook. I had made up my mind. I was no longer prepared to continually battle in the way that I felt I had been with my weight.

I can't quite remember when the thought process clicked in to have surgery - if it was whilst in an unhappy marriage, or in response to another nasty comment which just stabbed into me again. Or if it was the continual fluctuation in weight or the stomach ulcers which caused me so many issues... but something did click and when it did, it clicked firmly into place. It was a stark awakening. I realised that I am my own human. I own my own body. I make my own decisions. I am the one who decides if I feed myself or not. It is my body to work on, and my mind to manage. It is my life to achieve the best that I can. And that was that. My mind was made up. I was going to take full control of my weight and my life.

I went to seek guidance and support on the whole process, but I very quickly realised that there was not much out there, certainly nothing easy to find, nothing personable or relatable. I googled like a crazy lady and found all sorts of weird and wonderful stories and articles. There were books written by dieticians, who had never had surgery, let alone had what would be classed as having or have had a weight problem. Now don't get me wrong, they are professionals and every book has its place, yet for me, they were unrelatable as they hadn't actually been through the full surgery process. There were people who were trying to give advice and said that they had had surgery, yet actually hadn't, and then there was the hypno-band or something which I just laughed at and thought, if that really worked, there would be a queue around the block with thousands of us shouting *"hypno-band me up baby!"*.

Through the process of elimination, I found a private hospital where the same surgeon's name kept coming up as one of the best. Without telling a soul, I booked and attended a complimentary private appointment with him. I was a nervous wreck, slightly guarded through fear that he would be critical and judgemental. However, he was anything of the sort. He was relaxed, approachable, non-judgemental, detailed and highly knowledgeable. He answered all of my many questions and put my mind at ease.

However, despite his skills and knowledge, and two 30-minute appointments with a dietician, there was - and I feel to this day, there still is - minimal guidance out there outside of the medical information, unless you go onto a forum and publicly ask, and sometimes that guidance and those recommendations are a bit wild west, I only know that now having been through the full process and having maintained my weight loss for such a long time. It feels like there is nowhere you can turn to for answers to those private questions, where you can go away and read about them confidentially, nowhere to give you the amazing parts of the process, along with the hard truth - the rough with the smooth, the laughter with the tears; the actual lived experience.

There is nothing available to us by someone who has been through surgery to make us aware of the emotional rollercoaster of the whole process - not written by a dietician or jointly written by one. Nothing to describe how surgery positively affects your mind, your career, your health and how your surgery impacts your wider family. Nothing to highlight the potential pre and post-surgery problems you may face. We almost go into surgery semi-blind and certainly come out of the theatre completely bewildered with what may happen along the rest of our journey.

This is why, after over six successful years, I have decided to write my story and share many of my experiences with you, so that you can benefit from them and learn from them, to support your individual successes. And I can't wait to be a part of your journey.

You will join me as we head through my whole journey from start to finish. I will share with you things you can expect on your journey, things that take you by surprise and things you may not have considered - the laughter and the tears, the feelings you will feel and the unexpected amazing things to come.

I hate to think about the amount of money I have spent on a whole variety of weight loss clubs, diet pills, detox drinks, gym memberships, toning tables, running clubs, clothes, shoes, indigestion tablets, and never mind the emotional consumption of food and drink. I am not saying these tools don't work for some, they just didn't work for me in the long term. I imagine you may have felt the same at some point in your journey.

The thought of how much it might all add up to financially actually makes me feel a little bit sick. I imagine I could have paid for my surgery three times over. I sometimes wonder, if I had had my surgery years ago, could I have afforded to have the new car sooner? Talking about cars, can you imagine how much extra petrol we have paid to carry our extra weight around? I wonder if that is an actual thing? You know like taking extra luggage on a plane. I think it may well be.

At the time of writing this book, I am six years and eight months post-surgery and have successfully maintained a six-stone weight loss. It was through helping many other gastric surgery patients and/or their families, that I realised the same questions were asked and that there was no support book out there for our community. I can also relate to you, knowing the strength it takes to take care of yourself above anything and anyone else.

Depending on your current weight or surgery start weight, my weight loss may not sound like a lot to you. Then again, it might sound like lots or could be exactly the same as yours. All of our weight loss journeys are individual to us, as our bodies are all different. The journey of getting to the point where we have decided gastric surgery is the right thing for us to do is individual to us, however, we will certainly have some similarities. I am only 5ft tall. Six stone is a lot of weight for someone of my height to be carrying around as extra weight and a lot of weight to lose.

Often, the information I found available would speak to me as if I was, well, thick, which I am not, or as if I was lazy, which again, I am not. And recently, when I have worked with more and more people who are considering having or have had gastric surgery, I have realised, we - those of us who are considering having gastric surgery and those of us who have chosen to have gastric surgery - need something relatable, that is transparent and useful, providing information that can be accessed regularly and anywhere, as a supportive tool for each person individually.

This book is based on my own experiences and I am certain it will support you in making the best decisions for yourself. It will support you in owning your decision, the management of your surgery, and your journey as part of the ever-growing gastric surgery community.

I also write for everyone who has experienced conscious and unconscious bias towards our weight, or our decision to have elective gastric or bariatric surgery. We will have all experienced this in some shape or form and it can be crushing. This book is for you.

Having gastric surgery was 100% worth it. I do not regret it at all and would make the same decision if I was able to wind back the clock. It was the right thing for me to do.

I want everyone to know that we all have an incredible ability to achieve what we set our focus on, and often, it is our own and others' perceptions of us that can limit that. This book will support you to change that.

My aim is for you to find this book informative, fun and supportive and I am grateful for this opportunity. There is a journaling section for each chapter available at

www.gastricsurgerythelivedexperience.com

to support you with your success and I urge you to use it.

My name is Louise.

I have a Gastric Sleeve.

Welcome to our book. Gastric Surgery: The Lived Experience.

We are in this together.

Deciding is easy,

when your back is

against the wall

X

1

THE DECISION

Deciding to have weight loss surgery is not a quick and easy decision. You may say, I made my mind up really quickly, but when you look back, you will see that there was a long journey to get to that stage. We go through the process of trying a weight loss club one more time, a different one, and then, nope, we decide to return to the one with the best offer, or where we liked the lady, or where we lost 2lb more than the one we are currently at... sometimes we just go for the friends we have made. We hit the shakes hard one more time. I am sure many of you know the drill.

You may say things like *"I am big-boned"*, *"My weight matches my height"*, *"My hormones won't let me lose weight"*, or *"It runs in the family"*.

Come on, you can't say you haven't been there. I am sure we have all had a box of hard-boiled sweets full of sweetener, that makes you poo a week's worth in one day, or have had 'healthy' chocolate bars whilst eating bread that is wafer thin and a jacket spud no bigger than the size of your fist, or the diet meals that realistically only feed a two-year-old. I think I have actually done them all. And of course, they all work... for a short time, maybe a couple of years as you are invested, the momentum is there, you feel great, and then it all wears thin and back round you go again.

We may discuss having surgery with family or friends, tentatively at first, testing the water, before we dive in to tell them. Or we head online into a group and post anonymously if we don't want those who know us to be aware of what we are considering for fear of judgement and retribution.

We toil with the GP 4-stage process. We work out the figures to see if we are able to finance it ourselves or if we need financial support. Do we ask if the health insurance covers it? Is it worth spending, borrowing, waiting, having it in the UK or going abroad? So much to decide.

We have sleepless nights where we think about it and we eat, and eat a bit more, through worry or stress or anxiety, or quite simply through, *"f*ck it, I will probably have surgery anyway. I may as well eat it"*. Then we are cross with ourselves for eating, and eat because we are cross... Ah, the delightful cycle of being addicted to the habit of food, powered by emotions.

I had battled with my weight since that one incident when I was seven years old. Do I hold that one incident fully accountable? No, I don't. Do I think it was a driver over the path my life took, yes I do. Over the years my weight would fluctuate by up to seven stone. Due to this, I developed, amongst other things, anxiety, fear of what people may say, almost assuming they had said things when they hadn't, confidence issues, stomach ulcers, stretch marks, sore skin, embarrassing situations, along with feeling fabulous and sexy when I was at what I would call a 'happy weight' - when you have that feeling that you are on top of the world. Overall, it's been a right mix of emotions and weight over the years.

From that night, 30 years ago, when I was eating sausage, chips and beans for dinner, having fun with my friends, I was conscious that people were watching what I ate and what I looked like. Looking back, it hit me like an absolute steam train, sending a shockwave through my system of emotions I shouldn't have had at seven years old. Whatever happened that day made me also hate the taste and texture of sausages - weird, but true - and I didn't eat another sausage for over 20 years (no rude comments please) and if they were on the menu for school dinners, I used to throw them under the climbing apparatus so I wasn't *"encouraged"* to eat them by the dinner staff. It is incredible how one event can impact so many things. I point blank refuse to remain in any situation I do not feel comfortable in now, life goes by too quickly for that.

And at that moment, I learnt about sarcasm. I realised people could say things that sounded one way, almost nice, yet meant something completely different. I guess that one incident, without me realising it, created my weight story, it created an identity that I didn't have before, which is that I was bigger than my peers, and it created a belief that I ate more food than my peers. From there, I had times when I was slim or average weight and yet I was always self-conscious of everything I ate, drank and how I dressed. Without a doubt, that incident set my weight journey. I imagine you will have one too, something or someone that has impacted you so heavily it has contributed to the creation of your weight story.

The teenage years arrived and I attended a large all-girls school. It was hard going at times, yet fun at others. I have a mixture of memories, many that contain good friends and a lot of fun, nice teachers, who were still allowed to smoke in the staff room, now that does make me feel old. There were girls at school who were bigger, smaller, taller, and shorter, yet many girls were called fat or ugly, even when they weren't. Some were picked on for other things, like where they lived, their shoes, their style of skirt, the shape of their nose, lunchboxes, handwriting, and the list goes on. I don't think it was any different from so many other secondary schools. I can remember being picked on for my eyebrows - I hated plucking my eyebrows, yet today, they would have been the height of fashion, although typically, I now pluck them so probably not. When puberty hit, my boobs arrived quite literally overnight, and certainly without a boob job. I was more hourglass figure than shaped like a stick. If I am honest, I think I hid behind my boobs as my weight went up and down. My boobs have been blamed for so much, the poor things, as have my hips. By this point, my weight was now very much impacted by my emotional state and it fluctuated up and down with that.

The first time I went to a slimming club, I was 14. My mum took me. My brain was already conditioned into thinking I was overweight. Maybe I was, maybe I wasn't. I think I may have been, or certainly felt like I was, which is why I asked to go. At times I wasn't overweight, and at times I was overweight. Either way, the process of attending a slimming club told me that I was and that I needed external help. Looking back, what I really needed was what we all need - to be accepted and to be allowed to grow into an adult without the continual comments, however, this is life and this is what happens.

For teenagers, it is such an impressionable time and I have to question if it is ok for them to attend weight loss clubs. I know my mum was trying to support me and my request, and without a doubt, I would have said I felt fat or something along those lines and asked to go, but looking back, it is only with hindsight that I can now say that it wasn't right for me. I can remember my dad, committed to the cause, saying things like *"do you reckon cottage cheese on toast every day makes you lose weight?"* and me saying *"it will make people sick so, most likely, yes"* and us laughing about it. I will let you into a secret, we tried it and we quite liked it. Although I didn't share with my mum how I felt, I felt humiliated. Humiliation is something I have only shaken off in the last few years post-surgery, and I am grateful to my mum and dad for supporting me throughout the variety of different ways I have tried to lose and maintain my weight over the years.

I support weight loss clubs, I know they have a fundamentally positive impact on people. I lost 4 stones through one and worked for one for a while. I also feel that other things work, like shakes, and crikey we can say pretty much anything works when we put our mind to it, it is all dependent on each individual. However, for me, my weight came back on.

As I progressed to college, I came more into my own, I began to understand that your weight doesn't define your ability to succeed, however, I did begin to understand that your weight can define how people perceive you.

Everyone has an unconscious bias, which can affect those they come into contact with, without even consciously realising they are having an impact on someone. People would perceive me as lazy, despite at the age of 16, having a job where I got up at 5.30 am to work in a heart bypass ward two mornings a week as well as studying and working another two mornings a week as a waitress. They would perceive me as lazy despite babysitting until 1 am then being up early the next morning to head to college where I would do a full day, hand my work in and then head home to sort our animals. How do I know this? By their actions, their comments and their facial expressions. It is easy to spot. I bet they didn't express the same thoughts towards slim people. I know that you know exactly what I mean.

I had a good time at college, in fact, I had a great time at college. Yes, my weight went up and down, however, it didn't prevent me from having fun and laughing a lot.

I must tell you this story. When I was at college, I had a great friend who was the most fun you could ever expect to experience in a human, I am sure he had enough fun in him for two people. We would go out in my car and as we stopped at traffic lights, he would lean out the window and wave at people in the street whilst shouting a name like *"Sally, Sally, it's me, whooo hooo, Sally"* all the while smiling and waving. The number of people who would wave back was unbelievable before the penny dropped and they realised that their name wasn't actually Sally. That kind of silly fun is infectious and warming for the heart and soul. It has been people like that who have healed my wounds when I have been hurt by cutting comments and actions. And for those people, I will always be forever grateful.

Despite what many may think, my weight or my own perception of my weight didn't prevent me from having a boyfriend, nor did it prevent me from achieving well at college, or having a job and a good mix of friends. What my weight did do though was open me up to people saying, *"you can't play that part in the show, she isn't big"* or *"how did you manage to go out with him"* or not always be included in the group activities when I probably would have been, had I been slim.

Let's put this period of time into some perspective: I am 5ft tall and at the time I weighed ten stone. Yes, ten stone. Teenagers and adults can be cruel and sometimes I think oh well, that's all part of growing up. But, oh, how I longed to be ten stone years later. And it was certainly my self-perception, which all related back to that one play-date dinner.

I am sure you have had some of these experiences at different times in your life, maybe even today. It is cruel and crushing, and comments can be spiteful and cutting. People's tongues can be their strongest weapon. The thing is, without those comments, we wouldn't necessarily be here today. This wouldn't be our story. I wouldn't be sharing my journey with you and you wouldn't be on a similar journey too. We will all have our own story and without a doubt, there will be similar themes amongst many of us. The great thing is, with our surgery supporting us, we can achieve incredible things.

In my early 20s, I dropped out of uni, deciding it wasn't for me and within six months, my drive to experience new experiences and achieve as much as I could had kicked in, including the love of travel. I worked three jobs and saved up enough money to go backpacking, travelling to Australia via Singapore. It was only then that I really found what I would call my 'natural weight', a weight that I can happily stay at if I move regularly and eat well - and by that, I mean balancing food that is nutritious mixed with some foods that aren't. I feel I found a good balance during that time.

It was the first time that I felt truly at ease within my skin. Whether it was the new environment, new people or the fact I was having such a good time, I didn't have the chance to give my weight any thought, who knows? Maybe it was a mix of it all. This happened fairly quickly. I was in hot countries, moving daily, sightseeing, working, travelling to a new destination, swimming or carrying a huge backpack. It was a time that certainly impacted my future conscious and subconscious decisions, understanding that I was able to be physically lighter and mentally brighter and, although not always completely, I also found it easier to manage my mind and my weight when I was in a good place. I knew I felt happier when I felt lighter, however, I realised that I would always be an emotional eater and that has never left me.

So what do I classify as emotional eating? For me, it is eating if there is something to be celebrated, like a birthday, or something great has happened like a job promotion. It is also if I need comfort during a difficult time, like a breakup, an argument, a rough day, or simply being due on. It could be charged through one of my children having a bad day. Basically, if I was emotionally charged or triggered, I ate. Food has been emotionally linked throughout my life no matter which way I turned. I just hadn't spotted it until I travelled and had the space to really understand myself and become me. In the main, I would turn to and had a deep emotional love - and still do - of chocolate. I'm 100% addicted to it at times. However, the chocolate tasted different when I was abroad, which also supported me in understanding that I didn't need it and that it had become a habit often linked to my emotional state. I imagine you may have some of this emotional eating happening to you too - or have had it happen to you. It is a habit really. We are creatures of habit. And a habit can be the devil for many.

A habit that is detrimental to you can literally destroy you and becomes the normal thing to do. The habit can become an addiction. As an example; every time I walked into the kitchen, I would open '**the cupboard**' to take a look and if there was something I saw that I fancied eating, I would eat it. Every. Single. Time. For some people it is a cigarette with a cup of tea when they get up, for others, it is the Friday night beer which rolls across into the weekend and for some ends up starting on a Thursday. All of these actions are habits, which have effectively become 'the norm', however, they are an addiction which, over a sustained period of time, has negative impacting effects, such as weight gain, cancer and alcoholism. Perhaps slightly deep, however, it is useful to understand how these habits begin and how they can sabotage us. It is by understanding habits that we can begin to change them. I will come on to this throughout the following chapters.

In my late 20s, I had my first child. I gained a lot of weight, around seven stone. I had excessive nausea and vomiting bordering on what is known medically as hyperemesis gravidarum (HG) for the first six hours of every day from the moment I woke up I was sick. Basically, you just can't stop throwing up. I have absolutely no idea why just for that time frame, however, as soon as that subsided each day, I ate, and no doubt overate, to compensate. Looking back, I don't think I was overly happy with my environment and I feel that also played a part in that eating cycle. Although my firstborn weighed just over 7 lbs, I was left with seven stones of excess weight to do something with.

It was during this time that I met one of my most valuable friends. She has always accepted me for me and I have always accepted her for her, no matter what the life situation. She has never judged me on my weight, my life situation or on having surgery. She is extremely supportive of whatever I do and accepts me for being me. I sincerely hope you have one of those kinds of friends. If you do, treasure them. If you don't, you will. Yours will come along, give it time.

During the following decade, I was absolutely an emotional eater. Life was tricky, my then-husband would be away with work a lot, I was away from family juggling life as a busy mum and I would eat for all sorts of reasons. I also have Coeliac disease, which was diagnosed in my mid-30s. This definitely contributed to my emotional eating. Why? Well, with Coeliac disease, one of my symptoms is mild depression, which is very similar to PMS and eating when you are due on. I had also developed stomach ulcers through my weight fluctuation and my Coeliac disease, which again, without a doubt contributed to my weight. My weight would move up and down by five stones minimum, depending on how I was feeling, how well I was and what was happening around me. I would also have acid reflux, so I would eat more to try and settle my stomach. It was at the point of my coeliac diagnosis that my stomach ulcers were found through an endoscopy. Some of them were as large as the top of a pint glass.

So, if I could lose weight previously, what drove me to have surgery? It is quite simple really. I had had enough of yo-yo dieting and weight losses and gains and then finding my stomach ulcers. It was shortly after this that I began to consider surgery, thinking two birds and one stone. It was time to make a change for good. Take the stomach ulcers with the stomach.

You don't have
to do anything
alone,

I am here with you

x

2

WHY YOUR NEW BEGINNING STARTS

The only way you have got to the point of wanting to have gastric surgery, is that you have had enough. Like I had. You are at the end of feeling the way that you do. You have no doubt felt the way you have for many years. If you have already had surgery, you will absolutely be able to relate to this. You will have been at *"that"* point. The point where you just cannot continue in the way that you are. You do not want to continually think about food in the way that you do. To put it simply, you WANT to lose weight and FEEL GREAT for the long term.

It could be the feeling of being overweight, embarrassed, hot, cold, sweaty, or inferior. You may have areas of your body that get sore from chaffing, shoes that don't fit, and clothes shops that don't cater for you unless you want to wear sack-shaped clothes. Then there is fear of chairs that you won't fit in, chairs that might break, the list is endless. It could be the comments that people make, clothes that dig in, watches that don't fit, or feet that swell up. You may require an extended seatbelt on the aeroplane, cinema seats may be uncomfortable, you do not want to have a bath as it isn't actually big enough, having to sit in any chair when you are in a group and feel like people are sitting too close on either side of you - if you are anything like me, I used to find it dreadful. Like a living hell.

You may have fallen in love with someone you just can't tell due to fear of rejection, or putting up with people's comments regarding you being lazy or fat (I **absolutely** detest that word). You may have been in a toxic relationship, be that with a friend, romantic partner or family member, that for one reason or another, they put you down or encouraged you to eat. There are many people who encourage others to eat so do watch out for them, they are human sabotagers and more than likely fear your potential success.

You may have had your feelings assaulted, and you turn to food or drink, or both for emotional comfort. You may have experienced people thinking you aren't able to do a job or are not clever enough due to your weight. Their conscious and unconscious bias makes the decision for you.

I've been there, I hear you. My gosh, **I HEAR YOU** and I will always stand with you, strong, in that shared pain.

You may be fed up with what people say to you, the way that they say it or the way they react. It would be right for me to explain to you that this won't go away, sooooo many people always have an opinion on, well, anything they fancy really, and some just can't keep their opinions to themselves. However, the opinions that they have will change and you will begin to receive comments you never expected to hear. Depending on who you share what information with, everyone will still have an opinion, except rather than their opinion on you being overweight, their opinion will now be on your surgery, your weight loss and the new you. There will be people who have known you a long time and can't quite cope with the change, or feel threatened by your change. It is a bit weird. And if they didn't know you before surgery and had never seen you overweight, be ready for the wonderful comments you will receive, and you just don't know what to do with them.

So stay buckled up, because whether they are aware of your surgery or not, they will have an opinion and will be happy to give it to you. By telling you to buckle up, isn't to make you worry that everyone will have negative comments, absolutely far from it, you will receive so many positive comments, you won't actually know what to do with them.

It will be alien to you. You won't always know how to process the nice comments and feelings you receive and experience. This is something that we will cover in Chapter 22: Silver Coins. And if you are post-surgery, I am sure you can relate to this and know exactly what I mean. So for those of you yet to decide or yet to have your surgery, trust me when we say the amazing comments are on their way.

The good thing, no, the GREAT thing is, that now you have made the decision to either research surgery, have surgery, or have had your surgery, this really is the start of your new beginning, of you becoming your new you. If you have had your surgery and need a nudge to get you back on track for success, then this book really will support you to do that.

Weight loss surgery is an effective means of losing weight, however, it is a tool. The better you use your tool, the more successful the outcome. It may be that you have tried many methods of weight loss, and this is the area you are exploring or you have already made the decision, whichever it is, you do need to be mindful that gastric surgery is not a miracle cure.

Like all methods of weight control, it requires effort and commitment to yourself, to life changes to ensure successful and sustained weight loss, which will in turn improve your overall health. There will be changes to your lifestyle, your eating and drinking and your movement habits that will ensure your operation works as well as it can for you.

It is time to make yourself your number one priority, because, without you being your number one priority, you and all of your other priorities will suffer in the long run.

Are you ready? Let's get started on your new beginning.

From strong roots

grow trees that

beautifully blossom

X

3

GETTING YOUR FOUNDATIONS IN PLACE

A s adults, before we do anything, we research... or at least, we should.

If our child was going to a new school we would take a look on the website, speak to people we knew who had children there, go for a visit, and be nosey. If we were booking a holiday, we would take a look through the travel agent's websites, check out Tripadvisor, and social media groups, and perhaps speak to people who had been there on holiday themselves. If we were moving home, we would go and take a look at the area, view the property, usually more than once, and check out what the neighbours looked like.

We usually wouldn't make any of those decisions without doing our research and checking things out. Sometimes we don't agree with the information provided because we have had a different experience or we liked the area when we went to visit, or we know someone in the school we like, however, we make our decision on the information we find and the feelings we feel.

This is a normal process and one you shouldn't forget to do for your own surgery. I would say that this is as fundamental as following the guidelines post-surgery. And it doesn't mean the more you pay, the better the service or the less you pay the worse the service, do bear that in mind.

PRE-SURGERY

If you are Pre-Surgery, the first thing I recommend you do is research as much as you can. Set yourself a timeframe and really try to stick to it. Why? Because it will be the first part of training your brain to support the new you - learning to live within certain parameters will become your norm. Set yourself say 3-6 months, or a time frame that suits you, to do all of your checks and make your decision - it could even be one week, but make sure you do set that time frame and those parameters.

Firstly, I wholeheartedly recommend you speak to your GP or to your medical practitioner in the country you live in and ask for things to be documented on your record. A GP is a General

Medical Practitioner in the UK. If the first GP isn't supportive or informative, ask for another and see if they will support you. And, do you know what? If they aren't supportive or informative, that's ok, they are not experts in everything. Thank them for their time, appreciate that they have hundreds of patients to see, but every time you go, mention what you are seeking as that may be the final piece of the puzzle that triggers the Stage 3 process for you on that particular day.

Secondly, I recommend that you contact multiple private consultants alongside the GP conversations too. See if you can book a free or minimal-charge consultation in your home country or online in a country you are comfortable travelling to for surgery if you choose to travel. This will be hugely beneficial to you, it will give you a real feel for who you wish to carry out the operation on you.

Discuss which surgery they recommend for you, taking into consideration any and all other medical concerns you have, and listen. Listen hard to what they say, and make your notes so that you can compare conversations and guidance and make an informed decision.

You may have health insurance in place that will pay for private surgery, this is something that is still fairly new and we are only just starting to talk about it in the UK so it's worth exploring as people have accessed this in recent years.

Key questions to ask the medical team you see are:

1. What surgery do you recommend for me?
2. What is your surgery success rate of each particular surgery?
3. What is the weight loss success duration post-surgery?
4. What is the recovery time?
5. What is your pre-surgery procedure?
6. What is your follow-up procedure?
7. What implications may I face?
8. How long is the average time in the hospital?
9. Do I need to do a liver reduction diet?
10. How long is the expected recovery time?
11. What other things do I need to be aware of?
12. How will surgery impact any other medical conditions I have?

From these and any other questions you may have, and gathering your other research, you will be able to make as informed a decision as you can. Ultimately, your decision to go ahead with surgery will be based on which Consultant you feel is the best for you and/or if you want/or are able to go for private surgery.

If you are offered surgery on the NHS, you may not get a choice of surgeon. Therefore, ensure you do your due diligence into the surgeon offered as well as the hospital offered. When you come to research, look into each gastric surgery option that is available to you at that point in time as they do change, and sometimes surgeons may withdraw one. Options may include Gastric Sleeve, Gastric Bypass, Gastric Balloon, Gastric Band and so on. There are many to look at and choose from to suit you, and their popularity does change as does their availability.

My research included; internet research, conversations with my GP, private surgeon meetings, online forums and groups. I didn't know anyone who had openly had surgery to ask and there were no books like this. All the books I have seen over the years have been written by medical people who haven't actually had surgery. They provide their information based on medical experience rather than from the personal experience of a successful patient. They provide a very different viewpoint.

The surgeon said to me, the success of the surgery is measured upon the patient losing 50% of their excess body weight or reaching a Body Mass Index (BMI) of below 35. If you are unsure what your BMI is there are many online calculators you can access. However, although I look at my BMI from time to time, and by time to time, I mean yearly at the most. I haven't set my happy weight based on this alone. I am not sure if that is still the success measurement today, but that is what it was when I had my surgery, so it could be one of your questions when you are doing your research with each surgeon.

Use the following table or create your own version, to support your decision.

Research for success:

Surgery option	e.g. Gastric Sleeve			
Surgery Details	Removal of ¾ of the stomach to create a banana-shaped stomach.			
Which Hospital	Royal Hospital			
Which Surgeon	Mr Smith			
Pros	Removal of hunger hormone Restrictive stomach so weight gain is reduced Stomach is hard to "stretch"			
Cons	Can use "slider" foods Stomach can "stretch" if not looked after correctly Some people can suffer from reflux			
Outcome post-surgery	Average 50% of excess body weight lost			

The first time I met the gentleman who was to become my surgeon I had already done a fair amount of research on him, you could probably class me as a borderline stalker. I knew where he worked, when he worked there, and the weight loss surgery methods with which he worked. He seemed highly experienced and there were a number of good reviews on him. I really liked the fact that he also undertook other gastric surgery procedures, not just for weight loss.

I managed to get to speak to him before I booked in, he was easy to talk to and following that conversation, I booked in with his clinic. It was through this process and meeting the dietician he worked with before I properly met with him, that gave me the feeling I had picked the right team. She was kind, easy to talk to, non-judgmental, and non-patronising, yet firm and clear about the changes that would have to happen should I decide to have surgery. It was actually just what I needed and refreshing. The surgeon pretty much had the same character.

He was pleasant and attentive to what I was saying. He was clear that I wasn't the largest nor the smallest person he had operated on. He was detailed about the risks and the benefits, and he was kind with his manner and his time. He didn't charge for his consultations, which I feel is a huge win for anyone. He didn't pressure me to book immediately, or at all in fact, and he was available for me to ask questions once I had left his office, directly to himself if he was available or via his staff if he was busy. I still have the diagrams he drew in front of me today. By the time I left my second appointment with him, I knew he was the person to undertake my operation.

Now, you may say that he should be good because I chose to go down the private route, however, I can 100% guarantee you that not every surgeon behaves in that manner in the private sector. I left both meetings I had with him feeling that I was on the right track. My mind was made up. I was booking in.

I cannot stress to you enough how important it is to do all of your research correctly. Value your body and value yourself enough to do the research thoroughly. You are the most precious item you own.

In the run-up to having my surgery, I met with my surgeon the second time and asked him to go over everything we had discussed previously, which he did. He drew me a diagram of what would be happening to my stomach and where the incisions would be. As he drew the diagram, he said to me, *"Louise, this operation is not a miracle cure. It is elective and you are choosing to have it done. No matter what your weight, you have a choice. Once your stomach is operated on, it will become a tool for you to use, every day. Just like anything, if you use it well, it will do a good job for you. If you don't use your tool well, it won't. It is also important to take good care of your tool. If you don't, it won't function correctly, or it will become faulty and fail. So be wise, look after your new stomach, as your new tool, and it will do a good job for you."* Those words have stayed with me ever since. I am certain this one statement has played a huge part in my taking good care of my stomach and the success I have gone on to enjoy.

THE RISKS

I think it is useful for you to be aware of the surgery and post-surgery risks that were presented to me. I was made aware of them by my surgeon very clearly and if your surgeon or medical team don't make you aware of potential risks, then I would be asking why. In the UK, there are approximately 6000-7000 surgeries that take place each year. In the US, there are approximately 220,000 surgeries each year. Then we have those that take place in all of the other countries. I guesstimate that over half a million people each year have gastric surgery. How many have complications, it doesn't appear to be well published so I haven't been able to find the information to share with you, however, we know it does happen. Therefore it is key that you don't make your decision blindly.

The risks and complications that I was made aware of by the medical team were:

Operative risks

- Bleeding and bruising
- Staple line leak
- Deep Vein Thrombosis
- Pulmonary Embolism
- Chest Infection
- Wound Infection

Late complications

- Poor weight loss
- Weight regain after 2-3 years
- Gastro-oesophageal reflux
- Swallowing difficulties
- Stenosis of the sleeve
- Late leak from a staple line
- Adhesions with bowel obstruction
- Symptomatic gallstones

For me, I was so ready to have my surgery that the risks and complications didn't put me off, however, I did do all of my research and certainly prepared myself as best I could and looked after myself really well post-surgery. You have to work out for yourself what you are prepared to risk and what complications you are prepared to live with. For me, the benefits of not just weight loss far outweighed the risks and I was ready.

I do know of people who have had complications which include small infected wounds to the extreme complications of their internal organs stapled together by mistake. I know that is extreme, however, it does happen and is worth you making your choices with your eyes wide open.

If you have chosen a great medical team, if you have done all of the right preoperative preparation to ensure you support your medical team and your own body, and if you have put all of the postoperative care in place, most importantly, your own self-care, then you stand a very strong chance of not having any complications, like myself and thousands more. Always follow the advice of your medical team no matter what.

THE DECISION

Once you have completed all of your research, you will be able to review and reach a decision.

So what did I decide? Which surgery did I decide to go with?

I decided to go with a Gastric Sleeve. Now, don't get me wrong, having a gastric sleeve hasn't come without its challenges, which we will cover later, however, this was the right surgery for me at the time and over six years later, would be the one that I would choose again for myself.

My surgeon also offered it with a GaBP ring, also known as a Fobi ring, making the operation stronger and minimising the risk of regaining weight in the future. Not all surgeons provide this, but mine did and it was something I decided to have added to my gastric sleeve surgery. It isn't a band. It isn't inflatable. It doesn't move or stretch. It just sits around my sleeve, almost like a wide wedding ring.

The reason I chose to have a Gastric Sleeve with a supportive GaBP/Fobi ring was:

- The sleeve would remove the stomach ulcers I had.
- It would remove all of, or the best part of, the "hormone" that triggers hunger.
- The GaBP/Fobi ring would prevent my sleeve from stretching too much.

- It was the most successful surgery on the market at the time.
- I didn't want any part of my internal organs left inside unused and it removed the part of the stomach not needed.

Basically, I shouldn't be able to fit anything through my new stomach that is wider than a two-pence piece and still, to this day, I can't. That was my decision - a Gastric Sleeve with a supportive GaBP/Fobi ring, which I stuck to, and am very pleased with my outcome.

So take your time, do your research and make your decision from a knowledgeable standpoint. Take control of your destiny and choose the tool that is going to do a great job for you.

Prepare yourself
well to give the
future you
the best chance
of success

X

4

PREOPERATIVE PREPARATION PREVENTS...

P reparing yourself for your operation is key.

This is a huge, life-changing operation and something you should take seriously. At the end of the day, you have chosen to have this operation because you don't want to carry on at the weight you are, therefore, it is time for you to step up for yourself to ensure you are fully prepared so that you get the maximum benefit from your operation.

You wouldn't step out your front door to run a marathon without preparing unless you are an absolute lunatic. You wouldn't go on holiday without packing your case unless you are a nudist. You would ensure you have sorted your visas and passports, most likely had your legs shaved and been to your hair appointment. Why would you head into major surgery without preparing? That is exactly what my surgeon said to me, *"Prepare to be successful, Louise, and you will be"*.

- Prepare your mind
- Prepare your body
- Prepare your support network
- Prepare your fridge, freezer and cupboards
- Prepare your home
- Prepare your bag
- Prepare for ongoing maintenance of yourself
- Prepare for change
- Prepare for all eventualities
- Prepare to be successful and you will be.

If you are post-surgery, this section will really help support you to keep your focus or regain your focus if it has slipped.

PREPARING YOUR MIND

Ohhh, the wonderful internal computer we call our mind. It is one of the most powerful tools we have at our disposal. It can make and break us. It can support us to be successful and it can encourage us to fail. It is a tool for us to use to our benefit and it is time for our brain to now begin to support us correctly.

My guidance to you after all my time post-surgery is to begin to prepare your mind as soon as you can, even before you begin your Liver Reduction Diet (LRD). There is more detail on the LRD in Chapter 5. If you want to start to prepare, start today. And if you have had your surgery, keep strengthening your mind to build on all of the great preparation you did.

Begin to remove the *"one more won't hurt"* mentality, because it will. Begin to monitor emotional eating and find ways to occupy yourself or control your mind to process the emotions in a different way. Begin to be aware of the subconscious thoughts that can sabotage you, like your Negative Nelly - the one in your mind saying *"You look really big today"* as you look in the mirror (Negative Nelly giving us our nasty thoughts), or *"just eat it, no one is watching"* (Negatively Nelly giving us negatively encouraging thoughts). You get the drift.

Our mind is an incredible thing and I will share with you what I have done to keep my mind in check. Now, don't think I am a saint, I am absolutely not. What I have done is learnt how to control my mind to manage my new life as best I can.

I built up my internal mantras. This is something that many successful people do to ensure that they are focused on their own success. I realised that there was no point in reinventing the wheel, if it worked for them, it can work for me. I tell myself every single day "*I am happy and healthy and am making the best choices for myself*". I tell my body that I love it and that I am grateful for it. I have also extended this out to other areas of my life and feel that positive mantras really help you achieve the success you want. You may think that this sounds crazy, but I can assure you as crazy as it sounds, it works.

I began removing 'second helpings' and 'one more' of both food and drink. I removed eating in between meals unless it was a high protein intake as best I could. Again, I am not 100% a saint on this, however, just starting and then revamping whenever you feel bad habits are taking over, will certainly create a positive difference.

I began to not have a drink for 30 mins before or after a meal which supports the future new stomach. I prepared myself well as well as I could in advance for this action as it takes some practice. There is more on this in Chapter 8 - Learn The Lingo.

If you have already started any part of this process. Keep it up. It will be of huge benefit to you. Every time you feel yourself slipping, re-read this chapter. Remember why you manage your thoughts. Remember why you control your mind. Remember what it is you want to achieve. Keep at the front of your mind exactly how you want to feel.

Keep yourself in the game. Keep your focus on yourself. Do not let anyone distract you from your own success. No matter who they are.

PREPARING YOUR BODY

There are things that I wish someone had shared with me before surgery to go alongside the medical advice and help me prepare my body better in advance. To ensure you are as well prepared as you can be, I am going to share these things with you now.

You are going to have major surgery which will be life-changing and we wouldn't do anything else that was life-changing without preparing for it as best we could, especially if we know that the life-changing event is going to happen.

I was advised to walk for at least a mile every day post-surgery, literally from day one. So try and start now. As far ahead of surgery as you can. Get yourself into the habit of walking. If you already walk, add more time or distance to that walk. If you don't do any walking outside of your normal movement routine, then start. Build yourself up and get yourself into the habit of walking. Every step counts. I downloaded a distance app onto my phone which tracked my movement, eventually buying a smartwatch and getting savvier with different apps. I hadn't appreciated how good walking is for us and I regularly walk now, for exercise and for my mind. It is great for clearing and focusing the mind.

It was hugely key in my recovery and supported me post-operation. When I was in the hospital, on the first post-operative day, I was encouraged to get up and start walking. In fact, I was made to get up and walk, not physically made, but certainly heavily encouraged, so prepare yourself for that. The nurses had worked out that one mile was a certain number of laps of the ward floor and I had to build myself up to that point to be able to go home, so, very gently, with a little help, off I went. This wasn't up for discussion, this was an essential part of post-op recovery and supported the reduction of all sorts of post-op concerns, like deep vein thrombosis. When I think back, it is funny as the day before you are walking without thinking about it. Post-op, you are thinking about every single step. What I can tell you is that with every step, it gets easier, with every step, you become more confident, and with every step, you are one step closer to a full and successful recovery. So despite feeling fragile or excited on your run up to your surgery, get your bum out of that bed and get walking as soon as you can.

PREPARE YOUR SUPPORT NETWORK

You may or may not choose to tell people you are having surgery. Some people do and some people don't. I kept my support network very small at the beginning and I only told those I felt immediately needed to know. I told my mum, my dad, my grandma and my then-husband. That was it. I made the decision that absolutely no one else needed to know at that point in time. However, what I didn't prepare for was the drastic weight loss and people noticing quite so quickly. More on that later.

My mum and dad both had questions, my mum more than my dad, perhaps that's a female thing? Both were very supportive. My grandma just wanted to be sure my surgeon was qualified and not working at a "*back street chop shop*" - seriously that is what she said! My husband at the time didn't really have an opinion. If I am honest, our marriage had been difficult for a few years and we separated four months later, but that was already on the cards. Was it a driver in my operation? Quite possibly - most likely subconsciously, however, it wasn't anywhere close to being my main driving factor as we had separated a year before and despite trying again, things just weren't right.

My mum had previously supported my grandma through bowel cancer, and although not the same surgery, they were both well placed to advise how I may feel post-surgery and the best ways to support my recovery. My mum was an integral part of my recovery, both in the hospital and at home. She helped me wash and change in the hospital and she was a dab hand at seeking high-protein foods to support my recovery once I was home. My dad was equally useful but in a different way. He came to stay for the second-week post-op and, as a chef, he made me homemade, high-protein chicken consommé soup to support my recovery. You may not have this experience on hand to you so do self-prepare as much as you can. Super-markets sell high protein soups, consommé soup is a great one, or you could have a go at making some and freezing it beforehand.

And that was it. That was my network. I didn't tell anyone else. My children knew I was having an operation, but not what, and that was that. They were my key players. I am not going to even try to advise you on who you should or shouldn't tell. That is entirely down for you to decide. It is personal to each of us. Even today, I don't go around telling people unless it comes up in conversation somehow, it is now just me and my normal life and I approach it the same way as I would anything else, it is on a need-to-know basis, well until I shared my story in this book it was.

What I do want to share with you is that I have made and lost friends through this process. Perhaps some were jealous that I lost weight, perhaps they didn't like the fact that I have changed for what I feel is the better, or perhaps they were annoyed that I didn't include them in my initial process, who knows? Yes, I miss their friendship at times, however, if they responded in the way that they did, perhaps they were not true friends. Either way, I wish them well. At the end of the day, it is our bodies and our lives and we can choose what we share and with whom. I do suggest that you do have a small trusted support network, even if it is just one person, but again, that is entirely up to you.

PREPARE YOUR HOME

This process is almost cathartic. It is all part of *"out with the old and in with the new"*. Anything you feel you have that could sabotage you, hinder your progress or take you off track, get it gone or get it into a cupboard you vow to never, ever go into. Lock that bad boy and throw away the key.

My operation has impacted my whole family. We have gone from having a cupboard with crisps, chocolate and cereal bars in, basically full of crap to eat and fizz to drink - I am sure you know exactly what I mean or I am sure you have something similar - to having a small drawer with protein cereal bars in and the odd chocolate bar, plenty of fruit and veg and lovely high protein foods around. My change in mindset and eating has positively impacted everyone and for that, I am really grateful

Try and go through this process carefully. Go through things slowly and mindfully, and be measured. You don't want to panic anyone in your house either for example you do not want the children saying *"Lucy, have you seen what Mum has done now? She has binned all of the nice pack lunch crisps, we have to have air-fried root vegetables only!"* or *"Frankie, have you seen what Dad has done? He has put all of the chocolate spread in the bin, we have to have seeded bread with hummus on for breakfast!"* (Cue wailing and tantrums and being the worst/or best parent ever depending on how you look at it) You get the drift. This actually makes me laugh writing this and I can imagine it will have happened in some households, however, if you do things in a measured fashion, they will become positive habits and be accepted by all.

I began by looking at what was available for me in the house that I needed. I would recommend stocking up on high-protein soups, yoghurts, and milk powders and buying some peppermint tea to help with trapped wind post-surgery. Take a look at buying smaller bowls, plates and cups, to help with your visual hunger and mindset. Smaller storage pots are really useful to break down the portions correctly, and I removed things that made things just too tempting for me.

I prepared meals for the family in advance to take the pressure off of myself and anyone else, so that I could just chuck them in the oven.

I filled the car up with fuel and got up to date with the washing and ironing. Did a full shop. Basically, anything I could do to bring life right up to date to ease the pressure on the other side, I did it.

The other thing I recommend getting is a V-Pillow, or long, pregnancy-style pillow to support you in sleeping in the first couple of weeks. It definitely helped me as, post-surgery, I preferred to sleep slightly upright and when I felt I could lay down, it supported my tummy when I lay on my side. As time has progressed, and my weight has come off, there are still times when I pop a pillow or some of the duvet between my newfound knees. Ha, knees.

I also found it handy to have something I could push myself up on next to the bed for a few days, like a chest of drawers.

At the end of the day, as my daughter says, you do you because you know what you like, but please do go through this preparation exercise, it is very useful.

Without starting, there will be no successful future to enjoy

X

5

THE LIVER REDUCTION DIET (LRD)

WHAT IS IT?

The Liver Reduction Diet (LRD) is literally what it says on the tin. It is a diet designed to reduce the size of your liver so that your operation can be performed with less risk to you as I believe they have to slightly move your liver to get to everything they need to get to. Not every surgeon asks you to complete this, but from my experience, I would say that it not only reduces your liver, it also prepares you for the immediate post-operative stage and is a highly valuable two, three or four weeks to go through. Your medical team will advise you on how long they feel you need to be on the LRD so do heed the advice they give. The weeks may feel long, however, when you compare them to how many weeks you have been alive and how many weeks you will still be alive, they are nothing really.

The LRD is usually set to be followed for a certain amount of weeks leading up to your surgery date. I was advised that it would increase the chances of the surgery being completed laparoscopically (keyhole) as it helps the liver to shrink down. Being overweight causes our livers to become enlarged - something I was not aware of until my pre-op appointments. By following the LRD, your body reduces its glycogen stores. Glycogen is a form of sugar stored in the liver and muscles for energy. With each ounce of glycogen, the body stores 3-4 oz of water, so when you follow the LRD, which is low in starch and sugar, your body loses its glycogen stored and the water it is retaining with it. The liver reduces, as it has less glycogen and less water in it. Hence it is called the Liver Reduction Diet.

I feel the LRD is a key part of our preparation and is often underestimated, or I see people say *"Do I have to do the LRD? Having a few chocolates can't hurt, can it?"* or *"One last pizza"* whilst on the LRD. My thinking is, why risk your progress towards surgery or your own body during surgery? It is hugely important that you get yourself into the best shape possible for surgery.

My LRD was key for me. It allowed my liver to shrink so that the operation went ahead at a reduced risk laparoscopically (keyhole). It also meant that I was already beginning to prepare my body for what was to come. It enables you to begin to flush through solid food, preparing you for the liquid stage, and it also prepares you mentally. If you think the LRD is hard, then you need to double down and really focus on thinking it is easy, otherwise, the first few days post-op and the first six weeks post-op could be tricky for you and without thinking it could mean you make a mistake and put your body at risk.

What you want to achieve is naturally reaching for liquid and not thinking about food or chewing. Just a thought, you may want to brush your teeth and tongue more often too whilst on the LRD as your mouth can get a bit furry. It sounds horrible, yet it isn't, it is all part of the preparation for success and the more you can push forward in this phase, the easier the operation for the surgeon to undertake and the easier for you during the initial six weeks post-op will be.

When I began my LRD, the first few days were fairly easy, almost like a novelty. I kept the stomach and head hunger away by having warm milk rather than cold, and a sugar-free jelly in the evenings if I fancied a sweet treat. Then the head hunger and boredom hunger kicked in and it was time to really focus on why I was doing the LRD. So, to keep me occupied and away from any sort of food and drink, during the day I would keep myself busy, taking the children up to a local woods or beach and play park, and continually being out with them as much as I could. They were probably the fittest children around at the time with the amount I tried to keep active to stop my hands from putting food in my mouth. I would also paint my nails, over and over so that I couldn't eat as my nails were drying. It sounds bonkers now, but it's absolutely true. Anything that works for you is a bonus, so don't dismiss those easy wins in keeping yourself busy to ensure you achieve great things.

Equally, if you break your LRD for a moment or a day, don't panic, just get yourself back on track for the next day. Refocus and get yourself back in the game.

Interestingly, everyone's LRD is different. I was given two options to choose from. Option one was based on some very simple recipes and option two was based on what is referred to as the Milk Diet.

I thought long and hard about the two options I was given and decided to go with option two, the Milk Diet. Why? My rationale to myself was, if I am going to be on liquids for 3-6 weeks post-surgery, I might as well get used to it now. So that is what I did. It was based on some very simple rules to follow, which I will share with you. **I do want to stress that you must follow the LRD that is given to you by your own medical team**. We are all different, and all of our medical teams are different. Please follow what they advise directly to you.

So that you can see some examples of what you may be offered by your own medical team, here are both of the options I was provided with:

OPTION ONE - THE FOOD-BASED LRD

Here are some examples to give you an idea of what you may be given.

Breakfast

Small bowl (3-4 rounded tablespoons) of high-fibre cereal such as Weetabix, bran flakes, porridge or muesli - all sugar-free with skimmed or semi-skimmed milk from your allowance

Or

1 slice of wholemeal toast with sugar-free jam or marmalade

Lunch

1 slice of wholemeal bread or 2 crispbreads (no butter) with

50g/2oz of lean meat, chicken or fish or

25g/1oz of cheese or

2 eggs boiled or poached

2 handfuls of salad or vegetables

Dinner

50g/2oz of lean meat, chicken or fish or

25g/1oz of cheese,

2 eggs, or

75g/3oz of tofu or quorn

With

1 small potato or 2 tablespoons of cooked pasta or rice

4 handfuls of vegetables - non-starchy, so avoid root vegetables, peas and sweetcorn.

Across each day you could also add in

An allowance of ⅓ pint of skimmed or semi-skimmed milk (158 millilitres) for use in drinks and cereal

2 portions of fruit

1 low-fat, sugar-free natural plain yoghurt or

Sugar-free fruit yoghurt or

Exchange the yoghurt for another ⅓ pint of milk (158 millilitres)

2 litres of any sugar-free fluid a day of fewer than 7 calories per 100ml.

Tap water or bottled plain water

Tea and Coffee

Stock cube in hot water - 1 cup per day. Something like oxo or Bovril.

Squash with no sugar, fructose, sucrose, sorbitol or fruit juice.

You could add in:

Herbs and spices

Balsamic and other kinds of vinegar, mustard, stock cubes, tinned tomatoes and passata.

You could also make a soup from the stock cubes and vegetables from the following: Broccoli, cauliflower, cabbage, kale, tomatoes, mushrooms, sprouts, courgettes, leeks and celery.

OPTION TWO - THE MILK-BASED LRD (MILK DIET)

On the milk-based LRD the guidance for my daily intake consisted of;

4 pints of semi-skimmed milk (2.3 litres) - I could drink this warm or cold and use it in milky coffees.

2 pints of other low-calorie fluids (1.15 litres)

1 salty drink like a stock cube, Bovril or marmite stirred through hot water

1 portion of sugar-free jelly

Other fluids which I could have were:

2 pints of other drink (1.15 litres) in addition to your milk allowance, all of these must be sugar-free and contain less than 7 calories per 100ml

Tap water or bottled plain water

Tea and Coffee including herbal or fruit teas with no added sugar

Stock cube in hot water - 1 cup per day. Again like oxo or Bovril.

Squash with no sugar, fructose, sucrose, sorbitol or fruit juice.

My milk and fluids could be had at breakfast, lunch and dinner or divided up throughout the day e.g. ⅓ pint of milk (158 millilitres) 12 times a day.

And that's it. They were my two options.

The most restricted choices I had ever had in my life. I thought long and hard and weighed up all of the pros and cons of each and came to my decision. If I was going for it, I was *going* for it. I chose option two.

I felt it was the easiest option to manage inside and outside of the house. It meant that I could focus on my family and my job and prepare myself for surgery in other ways, such as mentally by starting my walking, rather than using the time worrying about measuring food.

For me, it worked really well. I could meet friends for a coffee and order a semi-skimmed latte and they would be none the wiser that I was on the LRD. I could go to work and 'forget' my lunch if anyone noticed I wasn't eating, and have a hot drink.

Interestingly, when I was diagnosed as a Coeliac in my mid-30s, the consultant said to me, *"Louise, if you really can't find anything to eat when you are out and about, remember a pint of milk has all of the nutrients you need, and you can nearly always find milk, or order a hot milky drink".* And he was right, you can pretty much always find milk of some sort and there are loads of kinds of milk to choose from now.

All of those reasons were really key for me in choosing option two for my LRD. It allowed me the opportunity to ensure that it was as easy and smooth as it possibly could be.

During my two weeks on the LRD, I lost 14 lbs. I felt lighter and brighter and almost cleansed inside. It had certainly kicked my cravings and habits to the curb and set me up for the best possible surgery and post-surgery success that I could have hoped for.

Occasionally, I go back to my own version of the LRD as a 'reset', especially where habits have crept back in that I don't want to continue - post-Christmas or birthdays, those sorts of times. I find it works well. Does it *"reset my stomach"?* It possibly reduces the size if there is any stretching, however, it certainly resets my mindset which definitely helps and that is what I use it for.

So whatever your medical team asks you to follow, or whatever options they provide for you to choose from, choose the option that a) suits you best and b) will set you up for the best possible chance of long-term success.

Please try and remember, there are over 250,000 people across the world going through this process each year. You are not alone.

Whatever your
decision,
wholeheartedly
believe in yourself

X

6

THE OPERATION DATE IS SET

Well that's it, your date is set and you are preparing your body with your LRD or other guidance. You will be feeling nervous at times, then excited, then unsure, then very sure, and then unsure again, the list is endless and the feelings and emotions will come and go.

You will begin to prepare and no doubt will have shaved your body to within an inch of its life, and possibly been and had your hair done, just as if you were going on holiday. You will have had your "last meal" before your LRD, and now it is time. It is time to get your game face on and be as ready as you can be.

So what will you need to take with you? Well, you will need a hospital bag, which will include everything you need for at least one overnight stay. I stayed two nights so I would recommend you pack a little extra. If you have been advised you will stay two nights, pack for three just in case.

I would highly recommend that you pack the following:

- Wash items, including a flannel in case you can't shower,
- A towel you like, you may feel fragile and will want a towel you like to use. It sounds weird but it is comforting,
- Easy knickers/pants that won't press on your tummy,
- A loose-fitting dress or t-shirt and bottoms, that won't press on your tummy,
- Easy to put on shoes, like sliders, sandals or easy to put on trainers as you won't be able to bend immediately. These may need to be closed toed so check with your hospital,
- Clothes that are comfortable for you to walk around the ward in. Short sleeves are best if you are on a drip,
- Hairbrush and products,
- Toothbrush and paste,
- Dressing gown,

- Hair dryer if you use one, be aware that you may not be able to dry your hair easily immediately after surgery, depending on how you feel lifting your arms up,
- A magazine, book or kindle, although you will may sleepy post anaesthetic,
- A phone charger, plug and long USB cable,
- Earphones,
- A portable device like an iPad or laptop, if you have one, to watch movies depending on how long you are in for or when travelling,
- Plug adaptor if you are having your surgery abroad,
- A Soft Pillow - I would recommend putting a soft pillow in the car for your journey home so that you can put it across your tummy and chest and under your seatbelt.

Before you know it, you are on your way to join everyone in the gastric surgery community. This is it, this is what you have researched, chosen to do and prepared yourself for. This is the last day of the old version of you. The new version is about to be born.

I chose to go to the hospital on my own. I went in a taxi at 6 am and I was quite happy with my decision. Why was I happy? Because I didn't want anything to change my mind. I didn't want an argument with my then-husband to cause me any stress. I wanted it to be an easy process. You will choose what is right for you and make sure you do. Don't let anyone convince you otherwise. If you want someone with you, ask them and take them, but remember it is your choice.

When I arrived at the hospital, I was asked to head to the ward. The team welcomed me. I was surprised to learn that I wasn't the only one having surgery that day and have, in fact, stayed in contact with others who also had surgery on that day, which is nice. These were a mix of NHS and Private patients. There were six of us and it was really nice to know that we were in it together. In catching up afterwards, we all felt that there was a lack of nitty-gritty information. That real sense of not knowing the lived experience. Which was a shame, however, it was what it was and is once of the reasons I want to support as many people as I can.

The nurses took us all to our own areas and I unpacked the items I needed to and got changed into my gown. The surgical team came to see me, which involved my surgeon, nurses, anaesthetist and dietician. I was taken through the process again, checked over and my time was set. I was the second to go down to the operating theatre. I was ready.

Now, I will be very honest with you, when I was in the room alone after the medical team had been and gone, I had a wobble. I suddenly thought what am I actually doing? Why have I chosen to do this? What about if I head back to a slimming group? Do a meal plan? Have my mouth wired shut? Is that even an actual thing? I really hope not, it sounds awful thinking about it.

And I cried. I really cried. The whole body jerking, lip wobbling, chest heaving, loud noise type of crying. I cried for the times I had struggled over the years, for the humiliation I had faced, for the nasty comments, direct and indirect, for the feelings I had had including no self-worth, or for being overconfident to try and hide my feelings of shame. And I let the tears flow. In fact, they are flowing now, over six and a half years later as I share that with you because I have never shared that with anyone. Blinking Nora, did I cry. I cried for the seven-year-old girl having dinner with her friend, for the school girl who wasn't invited to town shopping, for the teenager at college who had to stand in the canteen as others loudly questioned why my boyfriend went out with me. I cried for the pregnant woman sitting in a paddling pool trying to cool down, for the woman who wanted to wear strappy dresses and shorts in the summer, for the girl who had had all sorts of obscenities thrown her way - you know the ones, I am not going to give them air time - along with the comments like *"are you eating again?"* and *"don't you think you have had enough?"*. The tears flowed and at that moment I mourned years' worth of instances.

I haven't cried for that girl again, the old version of me, until today. Do you know why I am crying now recounting those feelings and thoughts and memories? I am crying for all of us. All of us who have been 'through it'. We know. We hear each other. The tears stopped then, just as they have again now. They just naturally stopped. By crying like that, I released all of the emotions I had been holding in and perhaps you will do too, maybe before, maybe after surgery. I want you to know that all of your feelings are valid, they are all part of your story. Release your feelings and say thanks to yourself for getting you through all of those times when you could have easily given up. Allow them to come, allow them to sit at peace with you.

And that was that. I ran out of tears. I looked at myself one last time in the full-length mirror, and I said *"thank you"* to my body for getting me where I was, in that hospital room and explained to myself that it was now my time to help my own body more than I ever had before.

When the nurse came to get me she asked if I was ok, I said yes, I was. She knew. She had seen it before. She held my hand as we walked towards the theatre and she said to me, "*You are going to be ok. If you have done as you have been advised and you continue to look after yourself after surgery, you will feel like a new woman in no time*" without realising it then and looking back now, she was right, I did.

When I came round, I felt a mixture of relief - I made it - and some mild pain - more discomfort than anything and slightly all over the place due to the anaesthetic - and I fell back to sleep. Anaesthetic can be quite funny, it can make you feel like you are dreaming, and you can have a wonderful conversation with the theatre staff as you are coming around. It can also make you feel groggy and quite emotional too. My now husband had a lovely conversation with his medical team after an operation on his knee about playing cricket. He damaged his knee playing rugby, nothing to do with cricket. I once had a conversation after an anaesthetic about being at a festival and asked the nurses why they weren't dancing. Go figure.

Something I didn't comprehend before is that the medical team have a complex job to do, so although I could have slept some more, I was woken up to have a small drink and to stand up. "*Stand up?*" I asked as if the nurse had just asked me to run a marathon. I explained I couldn't possibly stand up! The nurse laughed and said, "*Louise, you're not only going to stand up, but you are also coming for a walk with me*". I must have sounded like a right primadonna - "*I can't possibly stand up or walk.*" Funny, now as I recall it, however at the time I clearly sounded like a right plonker.

Slowly and gently, she got me up. Don't get me wrong, she was firm, and rightly so - had it been left down to me, I would have laid there dozing on and off. She disconnected everything, took all probes and wires off of me and took me for a walk to the nurse's desk and back. Slowly but surely, we walked. "*Now then,*" she said, "*that's good. Later we are going to ask you to walk to those doors and back*" - those doors looked like they were miles away. And as we walked back to my room she said, "*and then you will do your first mile*". Despite walking a lot pre-surgery, I am sure you can imagine my response. Those of you who have had surgery will know laughing is slightly off the agenda for a few days, and so is coughing and blowing your nose. So I made a weird "*ha, ha, ha*" sound. She quickly said, "*I'm not joking, and you will be able to do it, have belief in yourself, Louise*". Again, she was right, despite at times feeling pretty rubbish, I did as I was told and by the morning of day three when I went home, I could walk my mile, slowly, yet surely, and with ease.

The first night in the hospital was ok, I was a little teary, most likely from the anaesthetic yet also excited for my new future. There were nerves that still floated around and the odd time I woke up, I did have a moment where I thought what on Earth have I done? I don't think I am alone in those feelings. I am sure those of you you who have had surgery would have felt something similar and if you are yet to have surgery, be aware that a whole variety of feelings will come and go. I sipped my 25ml and slept off the anaesthetic. The next day, I was really fortunate that my mum came in to help me wash. I felt much better after having a wash and getting changed. I know I am lucky to have had that help and to put this into perspective, we live 100 miles away from each other, so we had planned it as she wouldn't have been able to just pop down the road. For those of you who may not have any support, take your time and do things slowly and carefully. You will feel a lot better after having that first wash.

I was sore and tender and I did have some trapped wind from the operation where they effectively inflate your insides so that they can work on you. The walking definitely helped with that, as did some peppermint tea and I tried to move my arms as much as I felt comfortable with. I am sure that peppermint tea is a bit of a placebo, I really can't work out how it helps with air trapped in your body.

WHAT DIDN'T GO SO WELL?

It wouldn't be right if I didn't share as much as I can with you. Not every operation goes completely swimmingly. For me, it certainly went as well as it could do internally and I had no complications whatsoever. However, I did have things that happened that you could see externally. Although these were not horrendous, they were uncomfortable and some of them were noticed by other people.

I suffered a lot of bruising - my arms, hands and tummy mainly - to the point I actually had someone approach me at work a few weeks later to ask if I needed confidential help, which I must stress, I didn't, however, that gives you an idea of how much bruising I had. My bruising went every colour you can imagine from purple to green, to black, to yellow and it was extensive. My arms and hands suffered the most. My tummy did have bruising, however, I expected some. My arms and hands were definitely from the needles pre, during and post-surgery. I don't feel anyone was overly rough with their practice, I think it was just unfortunate and I bruised easily which certainly showed post-operation.

I was really groggy and slightly emotional from the anaesthetic when I came around. Again, common for some, but not for all. Everyone was kind and, looking back, I think it was also the emotion of going through the operation. I had an allergic reaction to the dressings that were used on my tummy. The dressings gave me blisters where the glue had been, and it was itchy. I hadn't had that before with any plasters. Again, not that common, but it happened so I am sharing it with you.

You will hear that others have experienced other situations with the surgery and post-surgery recovery, however, from those I have spoken to and the forums I am in, any major complications seem to be few and far between. I am grateful that it was just bruising and feeling uncomfortable and I am thankful that all of my pre-surgery preparation set me up for the best possible outcome, and I still do, to this day, thank the full medical team for looking after me so well.

And that was it. On the third day, I walked my ward mile with relative ease, I had been to the toilet, climbed some stairs and was discharged. I was collected and, as advised, used a pillow to go under the seat belt and over my tummy. And home I went to carry on my journey as the new me.

You are stronger
than you ever
believed was
possible

X

7

WHERE THE NEW YOU BEGINS

The change in your life is immediate, there is no doubt about that. You have gone from being able to down a pint of liquid with relative ease, to sipping on 25 ml of liquid over the course of an hour. Your LRD will have kick-started some weight loss, however, this is where your weight loss story really begins.

When I first went home, I felt really different, far more so than I thought I would. I was careful with my body in the first few weeks and my confidence grew each day so I could begin to do normal life things. I have since spoken with people who felt the same and others who sprang around the block the first-week post-surgery.

It was quite emotional leaving the ward and the safety of the nurses and doctors. You are literally walking through the doors to your new life, you feel all of the emotions that you can imagine. The journey home was fine. As mentioned, it was recommended to me by my grandma to have a pillow across my tummy, under the seat belt, which really helped and also provided a subconscious comfort to the journey home. The children were so excited to see me, yet cautious not to hurt mum with too tight hugs. They made me a cup of tea which I carefully sipped and it was then I decided I needed to tell them what my recovery would look like. They didn't question it, they simply accepted it and from there on in, at each stage, they would make a drink and give me 25 ml of it at a time until my capacity grew at each stage. Absolute angels.

One thing to consider having at home is liquid paracetamol, rather than tablets, should you need some for any pain relief. Your medical team may give you some, or recommend you buy some, however, in case they don't, it is worth getting so you can take the liquid with ease and without worry should you need pain relief.

When you are home, remember to take things easy. There are obviously still things we need to get on with, but remember what you have just been through and take it easy. Your body will really thank you for it and you will heal a lot quicker, rather than you trying to do too much and putting yourself at risk.

I slept sitting up, not fully upright, just on an angle, for the first few weeks. Sometimes I was on my side, but I was always slightly up. For me, this helped and I slept well. When I felt ready to lay down flat, I used the pillows again to support me.

Getting up can be a little tricky in the first week. I remembered a trick I had been taught when I had my C-Sections which was to... hmm how do I explain this? Ok, I will try. It was to raise one leg in the air, link your hands under that thigh, and then use the weight of your leg to lever yourself up with your arms as the pully. I hope I have explained that correctly. This takes the pressure off of your tummy. Another way is to roll onto your side and then push yourself up. This will help you stop putting too much strain on your insides.

You will have guidance from your medical team, surgeon and dietician on what to do and what will happen over the initial weeks, post-operation, however, I hope my experience gives you an idea. Some clinics now provide a call line or a support network, however again, often with people who are medical, rather than those who have been through the whole experience.

I must stress that I took each stage very carefully. I was very aware that I just had ¾ of my stomach removed and wanted it to heal well. I wanted to achieve the best outcome possible. I was also aware that this period of time was for supporting my mind - to help it adjust to managing my new life. From day one in the hospital, you will most likely be given an antacid like omeprazole or lansoprazole, or an equivalent. Omeprazole and lansoprazole are designed to reduce the amount of acid your stomach produces, helping it to heal after the operation. I continued to take them for two years, post-op. That was the advice I was given. There are a variety of different opinions on this, however, I followed the guidance of my medical team and GP. I do still have them to hand should I feel I need them. They all became part of the process. I set my alarm 30 minutes before I needed to get up, swallowed my tablet, and then when I did get up 30 minutes later, I could have my morning drink with ease and the tablet would have had time to work. I go through phases now of needing them, usually when I'm not looking after myself properly. I know people who have been on them for years and those who only needed them for 8 weeks. Remember not to compare yourself to others too much, follow your own medical guidance and listen to your own body.

Once home, Stage one began. For me, stage one was three weeks of liquids only, and this is where the high protein consommé soup, the milk and high protein milk powder came into their own. I also mixed this up with some sugar-free jelly and tried to stay on top of my water intake throughout the day to ensure I didn't become dehydrated. Some days, those three weeks seemed long and on other days, it felt like it was flying by. The key to any timeframe for your post-op recovery is that you stick to the guidance you are given and you don't try and cheat yourself out of the recovery time by doing things faster. You will only be cheating yourself in the long run and effectively not giving the large wound/scar time to heal. Remind yourself of all the preparation you have done to ensure you and your surgery achieve maximum success. You have just had major elective surgery, you wouldn't rush anything if you had a major operation to treat something like cancer, so please take your time to take care of yourself correctly.

These three weeks really taught me how to deal with and manage situations, like ensuring I didn't get dehydrated at work due to not being able to drink as much as quickly as before - a headache usually reminded me to drink more regularly. The LRD meant that I was already practised in sitting with others as they ate when I wasn't. I sat with my children as they ate their meals and I had my small bowl of liquid consommé or a drink. That process enabled me to get used to people eating around me whilst I was on my own merry journey, eating slowly and small.

It made me realise just how much rubbish I had consumed over the years that my body really didn't need, and it set my mind to achieve the best results I could.

I walked my mile every day and the children came with me when they fancied it. It was a novelty to them and they would usually want to come, walk or bike and scoot around me. The benefit of this? We talked, without any tech to take anyone's attention away. It was lovely and a real perk of that period of time. We have continued to walk as much as we can together ever since and without me realising it at the time, it 100% improved the relationship between us as mum and children. We noticed things in our area we hadn't noticed before, we walked new routes, we drove to new places to walk and no matter whether it was dry or raining, we walked, because mum had to. Without them realising, they were my absolute heroes during that period of time. They still are.

I managed to drive two weeks after my operation. My insurance company said as long as I felt I could drive and could carry out an emergency stop, I was covered. I did still place a small seatbelt cover over the diagonal strap which I felt was more gentle on my scars than the seatbelt on its own.

I went back to work 10 days after my operation. I was dropped off for the first few days and took things easily. They knew I had had a stomach operation, but not the full details. I didn't feel that they needed to know. I had booked the time off as annual leave in the quietest period of time at work. Everyone was very supportive and once the initial *"are you ok"* questions happened, it became yesterday's news.

Stage two arrived more quickly than I expected; this was three weeks of purée textured foods only. I have to say, I was slightly hesitant. It was thicker liquid in my mouth than I had become used to and I was wary of how my stomach would react. I had the feeling I should chew, but did not actually need to. I am pleased to say, my stomach reacted well and I enjoyed this stage as much as a grown adult could enjoy eating like a baby, although it was quite satisfying keeping the purée in the bowl level as I could as I scooped each teaspoon out. As I cooked for my family, I would blend down a portion for myself and would use the consommé my Dad had made as gravy. I had portioned the comsommé into ice-cube trays and bags to mix through anything puréed to ensure I was maximising protein.

At the end of these six weeks, I was feeling in a really great place. I was over three stones down. For someone who is 5ft, that is a fair amount of weight. Please do not relate that to you and your journey. You will be taller or shorter and weigh more or less than my starting weight, we are completely incomparable. What we do have in common is that we want to improve our own lives, and will be on a similar journey, which is what my surgery allowed me to do: go on my weight loss journey.

Week seven began with Stage three. Three weeks of soft-textured and minced foods only. Think thicker than purée, but not as thick as solid foods. I was still really mindful of having as much protein as I could. This was where I began to chew again properly and where the 20-20-20 rule began to be used. We look at the 20-20-20 rule in Chapter 8. I didn't always have enough in my mouth to chew lots, however, I was hugely mindful to make sure I did chew so as not to cause a blockage.

By the end of week nine, I had lost four stones.

Normal solid foods resumed at the beginning of week ten. Stage four is normal textured foods. NORMAL TEXTURED FOODS. Haha. When I think about it now, I was absolutely scared to death. I was scared I might eat the wrong thing - and yes, that happened - or that I would eat too quickly - yes that also happened. However, I survived. What definitely happened was that I benefited from the 20-20-20 rule and the 30-minute guidance, and the days where I stuck to these like glue, I had the best days and I still do. These rules are like second nature to me now. Both of these are covered in Chapter 8. I started to eat solid foods, concentrating on protein in each meal. I took things slowly and carefully and I have to say, I was delighted to be able to eat solid foods.

By the end of week 16, I had lost five stones. By the end of week 26, six months after my operation, I had lost seven stones.

When I look back, I don't think I had taken care of myself properly for years and during this time I really began to enjoy looking after myself as much as I had always looked after everyone else. Enjoy this time as best you can and really take the time to look after yourself.

FEELING FULL

Following surgery, we begin to feel full much quicker than we did ever before, which is obvious really as our stomachs are smaller. The 20-20-20 and 30-minute rules help with this to ensure we don't overfill too quickly and therefore don't get enough nutrients in. You will be using small side bowls and side plates and will most likely eat around half, depending on the food and for me, it also depends on my monthly cycle as my restriction seems to change with that too. The full feeling is different to how it has been before. You can slowly start to feel your new stomach filling, which, if you overate, would fill up so high it would more than likely make you feel or be sick. You get a feeling around the middle of your chest like pressure from the inside. That is the sign that you are full or certainly that you are almost full. It is at this point that you don't want to overdo anything, nor continue to the point where you are overeating, otherwise, you will either be in a fair amount of pain until your body can process the food, or you may be sick, or you may cause a blockage which may result in you feeling very unwell and also being sick, so do listen to your body as it does talk to you and guide you. Be your stomach's best friend forever.

I do want to note that, more recently, there are people who only use pre-made shakes for pretty much their whole post-operative recovery and for all meals post-surgery. I am on the fence about this. Yes, you can consume the protein you require in liquid form, however, you won't get the opportunity to learn how to think about high protein in foods or cook different high-protein options. I guess every tool has its place. I do use shakes if I am running late or need something on the go and haven't prepared well enough to take something with me, mainly because I am also a Coeliac and sometimes Gluten Free Foods which are high protein and easy for me to eat and digest are not always readily available, so will have a high nutrient shake. However, for me, having a shake for every meal isn't how I want to live as I enjoy the social aspect of meal times, whether that be in or out of the house.

Whatever you are guided to do, or decide to do, do it well. Invest in yourself. You are the only one of you that you have.

Become fluent
in your new
language of love

X

8

LEARN THE LINGO

Did you know that there is a particular language that comes with Gastric Surgery? If you are just starting to consider it, you will currently be thinking, *"What? A new language?"* Indeed, like any specialist area, there is new terminology to use and there are a few terms and sayings that I would like to introduce you to. If you are post-surgery, you will be fluent in these and depending on how far post-surgery you are, recapping these may nudge you into using them again. Interestingly, my husband, yes I have got married again, second time lucky hopefully, said that although he knew I followed a *'pattern'* he hadn't realised what they were until he read this chapter.

Like anything that is new to you, or that you have not had exposure to, there is language and terminology which is useful for you to learn ahead of your surgery, that will support you in your future success. It is just like learning any new language, it needs repetition to embed it, and for us, it will also go hand in hand with a physical process.

Understanding these will help you prepare and be a key tool towards your success. I still use many of them today and the ones I get forgetful about, I retrieve and revive when I need to.

Let's get started.

20-20-20

The 20-20-20 rule is crucial and will not only support your weight loss for the long term, but it also prevents you from eating too quickly, which could cause you problems. So what is the 20-20-20 rule?

The 20-20-20 rule is as follows:

Firstly, the size of the food that you put in your mouth has to be the same size as a 20 pence piece. Secondly, you have to chew that food 20 times before swallowing, and thirdly, you have to wait 20 seconds before you eat again. Creating the 20-20-20 rule.

Let's think about that again. Anything you put on a fork, spoon, or bite from something, e.g., a banana, has to be the same size as a 20-pence piece. You should chew it 20 times before swallowing and you should wait 20 seconds before putting any more food into your mouth and starting again.

In my experience, the 20-20-20 rule is an absolute game-changer. It is something that I recommend you practice **before** surgery if you can so that you can get used to what it feels like.

Your portion size is often determined by your eyes and as the amount you can actually fit into your mouth won't change, - you don't come out of surgery with a smaller mouth to match your smaller stomach, that would be weird - so it is something you have to condition your eyes, your mouth and your physical movement into adjusting to. I recommend that you train yourself to put your knife/fork/spoon/item of food down as you chew for 20 seconds, which will support you with waiting 20 seconds before you eat again.

Now, you may be reading this and your mind may still be thinking about the size of a 20-pence piece and thinking *"Is she serious? That's tiny."* Well, yes I am, and yes it is, and so will your stomach be and, in turn, so will you be. Ok, you won't be as tiny as a 20-pence piece, however, you are going to be a lot smaller than you are now so get used to thinking and working with small amounts and portions. Begin to retrain your brain.

You will find it odd at first. Everything will feel small, and so will you, soon enough. However, it is something you adjust to and once mastered, it is a rule that will serve you well.

You will spend your time counting to 20 over and over and almost missing any conversation at the table unless it involves a 20. Only joking, you won't count to 20 forever as you will have conditioned yourself to know what 20 chews and 20 seconds "feels" like.

Think of the 20-pence piece size as 3 dimensional, not flat, otherwise, you will only be eating wafer-thin food forever. Like a little cube no higher or wider or deeper than a 20-pence piece is wide.

30-MINUTE RULE

The 30-minute rule is another that will serve you really well. This one is a waiting game and again, once you get used to it, you will just do it naturally. In fact, the second part of the 30-minute rule is really important if you are wanting to look after yourself correctly.

The 30-minute rule is where you do not have anything to drink for 30 minutes prior to eating or for 30 minutes after eating. This is to allow your stomach to be empty in readiness to receive food, to stop the liquid from attempting to push the food through too quickly and to prevent you from stretching your stomach. Allowing you to maintain your surgery success for as long as possible.

You will hear people say a variety of reasons why there is the 30-minute rule, however, that is essentially it.

So, let's think about this in practice. Before you eat anything, you now have to wait for 30 minutes after drinking.

If you are at home, as you plan your day - what you will have to eat and when - you will be able to work out the latest time you will be able to have a drink before each time you eat.

If you are out at a social event, you will be able to work out, when the last time of being able to have a full drink is by finding out what time the food will be served. And you will learn to gauge and manage these things well with practice. It is a trial-and-error process, but you will get there.

This isn't to say that you can't drink when eating, not at all, although that will be sips rather than gulps. It is to support these reasons:

- Your stomach will be empty and ready to receive food without over-stretching it through liquid and food together.
- You will be able to eat your maximum nutritious food rather than liquid taking up the space the food needs.
- You don't want the drink to push the food through your stomach too quickly as it could cause you to "dump" and no, I don't mean have a poo. We will come on to what dumping is later in this chapter.

Again, everyone will have an opinion on this, however, the most successful people I know post-surgery also maintain this rule as best they can, as do I.

I have come up with strategies to do this in social situations which I will share with you to begin to build up your own resilient tactics because you can bet your last pound that everyone you are out with heads to the bar or orders a drink from waiting staff to go with dinner. People will fill up glasses in the run-up to the food arriving, without you even registering it.

- I only order one drink before dinner and drink this slowly, socialising more than drinking.
- If I don't want to drink alcohol, yet feel peer pressure, I will ask the bar person to make my soft drink look like a gin and tonic with ice and lemon. I don't waste any money on expensive alcoholic drinks to not drink them.
- I order my drink separately if I can, or my hubby will order and he knows exactly what to do.
- And finally, I have learnt to say "no, thank you" to another drink.

Some of you may have thought of number four already - why not just say no, however not everyone is ready to say no thank you and deal with the peer pressure and comments at the beginning. Oddly, if you are only drinking soft drinks, they will accept the *"no, thank you"* straight away. It is when you are drinking alcohol that you will be questioned or encouraged to drink more, weird but true. Drinking seems to be the only socially acceptable form of a non-healthy habit that everyone is allowed to have an opinion on.

It is useful if you learn how to frame things with the people you are with. If you are happy to discuss your surgery, then they can freely know and that will close the conversation regarding drinking more. If you aren't and they don't know, then you will begin to build up your resilience and tactics to be able to manage any situation to your benefit. And that is the key part, it has to be to your benefit.

Whatever the tactics you build. That is the 30-minute rule. Use it to your advantage, to your benefit and to your success.

What tactics can you build to ensure you protect yourself?

	What tactics could I use?
1	
2	
3	
4	

DUMPING

No, this is not your uncouth teenager saying they need the toilet. This is not about you needing a poo either.

WHAT IS DUMPING?

Dumping, or dumping syndrome, is a situation you may experience where foods that you have eaten are too high in sugar, like ice cream, sugary sweets, full sugar jelly, some fruits, custard and even some heavy starches as they move from your stomach to your small bowel too quickly after you eat. It can also be referred to as rapid gastric emptying, however, people in the Gastric Surgery world know it as "*dumping*".

Like anything, not everyone experiences dumping, but it is useful for you to be aware of it, what causes it, what you can do to support yourself if it does happen and what you can do to prevent it.

Let's take a look at this in more detail as it is really key that you are aware of this process due to the side effects it can have. Foods that go through your stomach too quickly, that are specifically too high in sugar or processed carbohydrates, dump into your small bowel rather than trickle through, causing the body to react to that food or drink in a specific way, and causing the feeling that dumping does. Your small bowel senses that the food or drink is too concentrated in sugar and releases your gut hormones. Your body then responds appropriately to deal with what it has received. This triggers the dumping feelings.

WHAT DOES IT FEEL LIKE?

Well, it isn't nice. The first time I dumped, I was three months post-surgery and had two tablespoons of vanilla ice cream. It came on quickly and I began sweating, my heart rate went up, which made me feel like I was going to pass out, and actually think I would have, had I not put a cold wet flannel down my neck quickly. It was painful, which was my bowel reacting to what it had received, and it made me need the toilet really quickly. I suppose it actually does make you need a dump. It is like everything goes into overdrive and your body empties itself out in any way that it can. You may even be sick.

It can happen quickly, so within 10-30 minutes after eating or drinking, and it can also kick in 1-3 hours later, with slightly different symptoms. I have also experienced this, after eating a mince pie. It was about two hours after and I felt restless, had stomach pains, my temperature raised, I started to sweat and I just felt generally not right, then I needed the toilet, and quickly.

Typical symptoms of early dumping are;

- Sweating.
- Feeling faint or actually fainting.
- Feeling and/or being sick.

- Heart palpitations and rapid heartbeat.
- Feeling uncomfortable and restless.
- Bloating.
- Stomach and bowel cramps and pain.
- An overwhelming urge to lie down, possibly even sleep.
- Needing the toilet immediately.

As you can see, it isn't nice, and the 30-minute rule post-eating certainly helps with supporting you to ensure you don't dump. If it does happen to you, remember, it doesn't last forever. If you are happy to tell someone, then do, in case you faint. I have fainted twice, once in the early days as I had no idea dumping was a 'thing' and secondly by accident, which I will share with you later, so please do ensure you know what to do for yourself should it kick in, especially if you are out at a social situation or alone.

Late dumping can include the above, however, can also present itself as;

- Tremors and shakes.
- Feeling unhappy or restless for absolutely no reason.
- Feeling very tired suddenly.
- Fainting.

Dumping can be very distressing and can wipe your day or evening out. It is rare, but it does happen so better to be forewarned so you can be forearmed.

It is also really useful to work out which foods may make your body dump so that you can be aware of them in the future.

Make a note here. What foods do you enjoy that you need to be aware of that may make you dump?

	Foods to be aware of
1	
2	
3	
4	
5	
6	

There is a drink that makes me 'dump' really quickly and that is fruit cider. I learnt that the hard way and it was completely unexpected. I just wasn't thinking about what was in the drink, however, in hindsight, makes complete sense.

We headed off to the coast with the children for a week away and without thinking, I ordered a fruit cider. *"Ooohhh, I thought, I haven't had one of those in years"*. I poured the lovely pink liquid over the ice. Refreshing, I thought, for a nice sunny day. And it was. Until I began to feel unwell and realised pretty quickly that I was heading into a sugar dump, and it was happening fast.

My husband was down on the beach with the children, just slightly out of earshot so I text him for help. I literally wrote *"sugar dump, come now, toilets"* and I went. Walking as fast as I could, breaking out into the odd jogging step as I aimed for the toilets. I felt sick and knew my body was ready to teach me a hard lesson. I just made it. I didn't say which toilets and after making sure the children were all safe, he found me passed out, with my head resting on the toilet paper holder. We still laugh as people probably thought I was drunk and that he was the 'poor dad' with the 'drunk wife' looking after the kids. Fruit cider, in fact, any sort of cider is now on my dumping list and something I steer very clear of.

It is also really useful to make a note of those that have made you dump, should it happen to you.

As an example, I am really wary of ice cream. I still have ice cream, I am just mindful of which brand, e.g. how high the sugar content is, and if I do have it, I only have a very small amount.

What foods did I eat which made me dump and what were my symptoms?

	What foods did I eat which made me dump?	What symptoms did I have?
e.g.	Vanilla ice cream	Sweating Feeling Faint Needing the toilet asap Stomach cramps
e.g.	Fruit Cider	All of them and passed out cold. Steer clear always!
1		
2		
3		
4		

SLIDER FOODS

"If it slides through your body, it rides on your body!"

You may or may not have heard of slider foods. I hadn't until after my surgery and I was genuinely like, what are they? Do they slide because they are slimy and slippery?

Slider foods are foods that you don't have to overly chew. They basically turn to mush or liquid in your mouth and slide down, they don't fill you up, which means that they just "slide" through your stomach. They are usually foods which have little or no nutritional value and we eat them because, well because we like eating them. Like chocolate, cake or crisps.

When I think back to the 20-20-20 rule, these foods don't need that rule. You don't need to chew them 20 times because they would have disintegrated in your mouth by that point. I bet you now begin to really concentrate on what you are eating, how long you chew it for, what texture it is in when you swallow, how you have to eat it and why you are eating it.

Slider foods are also commonly associated with dumping because they go through so easily and quickly. Whether it is from an immediate sugar perspective or a large volume of carbohydrates you are asking your body to deal with, they are usually found in someone's dumping list.

Slider foods reduce down to liquid or 'mush'. They move through your stomach easily, which means:

a) your body doesn't have to work to digest anything because this has pretty much all been done for you in the processing of making the food.

and

b) you can eat more and more of these foods really easily, absorbing hundreds of "empty" calories really quickly. Due to this, they can absolutely sabotage your weight loss and mindset as they are "*easy to eat*", so please get your slider radar tuned in and be ready to realise when you are eating slider foods and the damage they can do.

Empty calories are the foods and drinks that are high in calories, yet lack nutritional value. An example would be chocolate. Chocolate is a slider food because it melts in your mouth and turns to liquid and slides through. The WORST thing about slider foods, aside from the fact that they can make you dump, is that they are usually the foods we have previously thought of as "nice" and "*a treat*" or we have been addicted to them. I was absolutely a chocoholic before my operation and no doubt, I still am. I just have that addiction in check as my drive to maintain my successful weight loss outweighs any benefit from the addiction.

Slider foods can also be things like crisps. You can demolish a bag of crisps, maybe even two, without overly thinking about it, because they turn to mush as we eat them. Literally, turn to mush in our mouths.

Other slider foods could be;

- Cakes.
- Sweets.
- Milkshakes - be really careful of these bad boys and their sugar content.
- Biscuits and crackers.
- Yoghurts and mousse - you know the ones I mean, the high-sugar, high-calorie ones.
- Large quantities of pasta eaten quickly.
- Large quantities of rice eaten quickly.
- Large quantities of mashed potato eaten quickly.
- Alcohol.

In my life, slider foods are usually high-calorie, nutritionally useless foods such as chocolate, cakes and biscuits. Be aware of them and get your tactics in place to navigate yourself around them as best you can. If I buy them, I buy a small amount. I portion them out and set myself a limit of what I can have and when. If I do eat too many, well more fool me really because I am not looking after myself. So, when Saturday nights roll around and I would have sat and had a bowl of crisps watching a movie, I try and remind myself that it was habits like that which contributed to me having to have surgery in the first place, so I really try not to. It is sometimes still a battle of Negative Nelly and Positive Polly, where Negative Nelly would certainly allow and encourage me to fall into a habit of sabotage.

I also love chocolate like bees love nectar. I can actually inhale it so I have to be really careful because if I start, I really struggle to stop.

Prevention
is better than
cure

X

9

FOOD GETTING STUCK

Without a doubt, at some point you will experience what happens when your food gets stuck. If you follow the 20-20-20 rule religiously, this will reduce the chances of food getting stuck, lots, however, there may be the odd occasion that you rush, or forget, or you swallow something that your body has decided it just isn't going to want to go through your stomach.

I have experienced food getting stuck when I have done exactly that, I have rushed without thinking or swallowed a too-large piece of food by accident. However, I have occasionally had what I can only refer to as food tolerance changes. This is when I have previously been able to eat food and it will go down and stay down with no problem, then for some unknown reason, something changes with what my body will accept and it will go down and get stuck. Without rhyme or reason.

When food gets stuck, you will know really quickly. You will get a pain, mine is usually around my sternum, right in the middle of my chest and often up my backbone. They are the easiest ways to explain where the pain presents itself. With that pain, I get what some people refer to as **"Foamies"**, where my saliva is not able to go through the blockage and causes a foaming sensation in my mouth. It isn't nice and as you get to know your new body, you will know if something is stuck.

WHAT CAN YOU DO WHEN SOMETHING IS STUCK?

As always, please follow the advice of your own medical team. The advice I received from my medical team was to drink something fizzy and sugar-free to help break it down. They recommended something like sugar-free lemonade or sugar-free Coke/Pepsi. I have to say, my first go-to is Pepsi-Max, lemonade second, and diet Coke third. Why? For me, I feel that PepsiMax works best, and if I am not able to get any when I am out or don't have any in the house, then I go to the other two. There have been times when I haven't been able to get any of those and have had to leave my body to work through it on its own, which is painful and tiring.

Around four years post-surgery, there was a time when I had a blockage and couldn't get anything to work to unblock it. I called the ward where I was originally a patient to seek advice. I explained what I had tried and that I was now getting worried as it had been over 6 hours. The lovely nurse said not to worry, and to go and lie down, on my side, whichever side was most comfortable and to try and sleep it off and it would naturally work itself out. I was unsure, and I was really worried about what would happen if I fell asleep, but I did as I was told and by the morning it had indeed sorted itself out. It isn't a nice feeling so do reach out for support from someone you trust if you can. I like to have someone rub and pat my back, a bit like winding a baby. I find that really helps, even if it is just a placebo effect through feeling looked after.

WHAT GETS STUCK?

It is completely different for everyone and it does change. In the beginning, I really struggled with chicken, but now I can eat chicken well. Then I struggled with fish, which came out of the blue and it was that change which made me realise that my body may change what it will and won't tolerate. Currently, I really struggle with salad and minced beef. I have absolutely no idea why. I am not saying that they always get stuck, however, if something does, it is currently that. Fish is back on my menu and I find turkey mince easier to digest.

As for dry bread... Well, I may as well chuck a plug down my throat and hope for the best. Dry bread is my worst nightmare to the point where I refuse to eat it.

Sometimes, when I am chewing I just 'know' if the food in my mouth isn't going to go through. I can't explain it and perhaps you will also have that intuition. When I get that sense, I know that I have to spit the food out otherwise it will get stuck and I will most likely be sick. Strange, but true.

Food getting stuck may sound very traumatic and you may be thinking what on earth.... However, if you follow the guidelines, and look after yourself when you are eating, you will hardly experience this, if at all. If you have or do experience this, then you have some of my solid experiences to draw from that could help you.

WHAT CAUSES DISCOMFORT?

There are things that I don't seem to tolerate very well. They don't get stuck, however, they do cause me some discomfort. Hard crisps, you know the ones I mean, the posh ones, for me, they are unforgiving. My stomach doesn't seem to like too many nuts at once. I really like them and they are high in protein, so have a handful at a time or mixed through some yoghurt. Hard fruits can also cause discomfort.

There are also drinks that cause some discomfort. This is my body reminding me that drinks that are too acidic, like fruit juices and some alcohol, are not kind to my internal system.

This may be the chapter that you want to share with others, especially those close to you or in your household. Once I had shared these with those I lived with, it really helped them understand what they could do to support me. As an example, everyone slowed down eating to ensure I didn't feel like I was rushing, and from that, we chatted more at dinner. There are lots of huge pros to our new way of eating and our new lives, beyond just weight loss.

Maintain yourself
well and
your body will
look after you
in return

X

10

ONGOING MAINTENANCE FOR SUSTAINED SUCCESS

B eing aware of your own maintenance is key. I didn't appreciate the positive impact of ongoing maintenance at the beginning and when I was around three years post-op, I realised that my own maintenance was beginning to slip. That was a big lightning bolt to me.

It started because I realised that where I didn't feel hungry, I was going some days without eating well enough, living off of cups of tea and coffee, gabbing a protein bar or some rubbish that was quick and easy to eat, day after day. I was a busy single mum, my career was back on track, I was working hard in and outside of work and I was dating a lovely man. In fact, I think the only time I ate properly was when I saw him for a date as the rest of the time I focused on the children and my career. I became unwell, not overly, just run down. Cold Sores, spots, rough skin, hair struggling to maintain itself. Those sorts of things. This also tied in with a check-up with the GP, including my cervical screening appointment. This is my little nudge to remind you all to go and get your cervical check-up. The GP ran some blood tests and although the results were not awful, they came back to say, start looking after yourself again, please. So, I took a stock check on what I was doing to look after myself and got myself back on track. Not just weight loss-wise, but holistic health-wise too.

To get my overall health back on track and to ensure I maintained my weight loss, I refreshed the following:

- Prioritised protein. If not in each meal, certainly across my day and week. Including milk and yoghurts.
- Livened up the food options in the house with fruit and veg that I could eat easily on the move.
- Managed slider foods. They sabotage you immediately.
- I got back to walking and other exercises, including Pilates.
- I made sure I body brushed, not just once a week.

- I bought myself a weekly pill box for my vitamins and minerals so I could keep proper track of what I was taking.
- I actually bought the vitamins and minerals to put in the new pill box.
- I bought a high protein, vitamin and mineral shake as a backup in case I found myself having a day where a meal wasn't possible until the evening.

All of these things really helped me to get back on track and bar a few odd tweaks I still maintain that level of looking after myself today. When you look at it, it isn't a lot really, we are just not always great at putting our needs first.

PROTEIN POWER

Why is protein important for your success and ongoing maintenance?

Protein is one of the key ingredients you will need to really take notice of. The guidance tells us we need approximately 0.75g of protein per 2.2 lbs or 1 kilo of our body weight a day.

Let's take a look at what that could mean for you.

The basic sum is 14 ÷ 2.2 x 0.75 = 4.77 = the protein intake for 14lbs of body weight.

According to NHS guidelines, and there are all sorts of guidelines out there, the protein requirement is as follows;

Stones	lbs	Kgs	Protein required 0.75g per 2.2lbs
1 stone	14lbs	6.35kg	4.77g
10 stones	140lbs	63.5kg	47.7g
15 stones	210lbs	95.2kg	71.5g
20 stones	280lbs	127kg	95.5g
30 stones	420lbs	190kg	143g

Now we know the maths, why do we need to ensure our diet is protein-rich? Protein provides a huge volume of benefits. I am no medical expert, but what I can share with you is what my medical team shared with me.

It is hugely beneficial to us that we focus on protein as the main part of our diet and add other ingredients alongside it to support that protein.

I enjoy the following proteins and they make up a large proportion of my food and drink intake a day.

- Eggs - in all shapes and forms, although I don't like greasy fried eggs any more.

- Cheese - all types.
- Milk - on its own, in drinks and low-sugar shakes.
- Chicken and turkey.
- Fish.
- Meat.
- Lentils, beans and pulses - I have really grown to love these and mix them through lots of dishes.
- Yoghurts.
- Nuts and seeds - particularly sprinkled on natural yoghurt with berries.
- Protein powder - including milk powders.
- Tofu.
- Tempeh.
- Quinoa. (I still can't say that properly)
- There are also many other great vegetarian and vegan options.

I researched high-protein vegetables and try to incorporate as many of those into my diet as I can such as broccoli and brussell sprouts. (pharp). Last night we had high-protein pasta, with turkey mince in a tomato-based sauce with courgettes, chopped brussell sprouts, onion and garlic, all mixed together with some grated cheese on top. You can be really innovative with how you raise your protein levels.

Protein supports your body in all manner of ways. It supports hair growth and muscle strength. It supports the body with wound healing, inside and out. Protein helps your body repair cells and make new ones, it speeds recovery post-exercise or injury, which is one of the reasons it is key in your post-surgery recovery as well.

You may hear people say or read that people often eat or drink protein to help them feel fuller for longer. We don't actually need to do that as we shouldn't feel hungry due to most of us having our hunger hormone removed from our stomachs, plus we now have a far reduced stomach size, however, do use protein in your diet to your benefit.

Remember, if you think you feel hungry, it could be dehydration.

VITAMINS AND MINERALS

In your pre and post-operation pack from your medical team, there should be guidance on which vitamins and minerals you will need alongside your food intake. In case there isn't, I do need to make it clear that I am not advising you, I am sharing with you what my medical team provided to me and what I do on a daily basis from working out what my body needs so that you can make your own informed decisions based on the guidance from your own medical team and from my experience and daily practice.

The guidance I was provided with was to take the following daily:

- A complete multivitamin and mineral - this could be prescribed by your GP such as Forceval, capsule or soluble, or if I was to swap to a supermarket brand, I was to take two tablets a day. I have to say, the prescribed ones made me feel sick so I found an over-the-counter one that didn't. Even now, if I take them on an empty stomach I can feel sick so I take mine in the evening before I fall asleep.
- A calcium tablet

And that was it. Despite all of the wonderful care I received, that was the main guidance on vitamins and minerals. I have spent time researching what else I need to support my body and maintain a healthy life specifically for me. There will absolutely be other advice out there, and hopefully, you will receive guidance from your medical team, however, this is what I have found works for me.

Alongside my multivitamins, I take;

- Vitamin D
- Vitamin B12
- Biotin to support my hair
- A perimenopausal vitamin as I have absolutely slipped into early perimenopause. Can this be attributed to weight loss? I don't think so, early perimenopause runs in the family. Then again, who knows?
- Collagen - I swap between liquid and tablet, as long as it is over 10,000mcg per serving
- A daily probiotic.

I find all of these support my body and I feel very well. Trial things for yourself to see what your body needs and what suits you. I always know if my body isn't getting what it needs as my energy and my hair are the first things to suffer.

BODY MAINTENANCE

Body Brushing

I body brushed R.E.L.I.G.I.O.U.S.L.Y for the first two years, and now body brush around three days a week. Why? I read that body brushing was supposed to be beneficial for the following reasons;

- Stimulates the lymphatic system.
- Supports the increase of circulation.
- Helps to break down cellulite.
- Exfoliates the skin.
- Supports the body to release toxins.

Whether it is or isn't actually beneficial, I don't know, but it is something I chose to do as part of my whole process and feel it has supported the firmness of my skin. Maybe it just invigorates me and gives me a bit of a workout in the shower. Either way, I feel it helps and that's also great for my mindset.

Exercise

Easy. Steady now. Don't go throwing the book down. DO NOT burn it to keep warm. Stay with me.

I have already shared with you the requirement to walk post-surgery and its benefits. I highly recommend it is something that you keep up with. If walking really isn't your thing, as you begin to lose weight and choose activities, it is key that you choose ones that you like, you want to do, and that you can sustain or swap around, so you continue to include some sort of exercise for the long term.

I still walk regularly and now include other activities across my week that I enjoy like swimming, strength and conditioning and dance fit. I have chosen to join a gym that provides a variety of options that I can drop in and out of and I see it as an ongoing investment in my physical and mental well-being. It helps to maintain my weight loss, supports my muscle and bone strength and supports my body as a female as each birthday passes. I go when I can - some weeks more regularly than others. The key is that I don't give up.

There are lots of gyms around where you can pay as you go, there are park gyms which are free, there are private classes, women-only gyms, men-only gyms, swimming classes and aqua fit, and then there is YouTube if you don't feel ready to join a gym.

If you haven't started doing any exercise, give something a go. There are plenty of options to choose from, just try them out. Everyone thinks people are worried about what everyone else thinks, and it is only when you realise that no one cares, or gives anyone any more than a brief thought, that you will overcome your worries and concentrate on doing things for you. I could suggest you try and take a friend, or go cold turkey on your own. Whatever you choose to do, make sure you have your journey of success at the front of your mind and you will find your groove, whether that is with exercise or not.

Alcohol

It is important to understand alcohol and its impact on someone who has had weight loss surgery.

When I was preparing for my surgery, my dietician explained to me how I would absorb alcohol quicker than I had before, due to having a smaller stomach, which seems obvious right, however, she said not everyone realises and can get themselves into some horrible situations. Imagine, if you were a lightweight with drinking before, you are a seriously cheap date now. I chatted with her about how I'd always had a low tolerance for alcohol. She made it really clear to be extra careful as I would feel the effects of alcohol a lot quicker, warning me that previous patients had experienced blacking out.

I have always had a low tolerance to alcohol, no matter what my weight was. I imagine if you asked anyone from my late teens and early 20s about me and alcohol, their keywords would be "lightweight" and "sick". I have never been a big drinker and that is possibly why my tolerance was low. Since surgery, I have really learnt how to manage alcohol for a variety of reasons.

- I don't need much to get drunk, maybe two to three drinks tops.
- It can cause stomach ulcers and I am really mindful I don't do anything to cause them again.
- It can cause acid reflux and that is something no one wants, nor wants to encourage.
- Alcohol can become a habit for us due to transfer addiction and it being a "slider food".
- It is empty calories and we have had our operation to ensure we lose weight, not gain, especially through empty, non-nutritious calories.
- It can cause you to experience dumping which is not a nice position to be in when you are drunk.

So how do I manage alcohol for my gastric sleeve?

I have learnt to drink long and slow. If I have a glass of wine, I have a small wine as a spritzer with sparkling water or soda and ice. If I have a Gin and Tonic, I ask for two tonics to the single shot of gin, and ice. If I have red wine, I add ice cubes. If I have a small beer, I add sugar-free lemonade as a shandy. There are lots of ways you can make your drinks last longer and have a slower impact and I am sure you will work things out to still have a drink if you enjoy having one, without any detrimental side effects.

I also use the same tactic I did before when I felt under peer pressure to drink in my late teens and early 20s, namely to ask the bar staff to make me a soft drink that looks like an alcoholic one - a mocktail, a slimline tonic with ice and a slice, no gin, sparkling water with ice and a slice, no-secco. There are plenty of non-alcohol style drinks available now too which there weren't back then. Some people drink to get drunk. I drink from a social perspective, but I can take it or leave it, the health of my stomach and my weight loss is more important to me.

You get the gist and you will work out your own success tactics when drinking alcohol, and no, I am not encouraging you to work out a tactic to get successfully drunk. I am encouraging you to work out a way to drink safely post-surgery that is for sure. Whatever you decide to do, make sure it is to support yourself and your weight loss surgery.

Fizz

You will hear many people ask about drinking fizzy drinks or you may have wondered if it is possible to drink fizzy and carbonated drinks post-surgery. The answer is absolutely not for the first few months post-surgery due to the pressure it could put on your incisions as your stomach will still be healing. There are other reasons to not drink very fizzy drinks. It can stretch your stomach, attribute to stomach ulcers, neither of which we want to happen. However, later on down the line, yes, it is possible to drink lightly fizzy or carbonated drinks, however, it isn't recommended for those and many other reasons. There are times when I may like a glass of white wine and soda, or a gin and tonic and always reduce the fizz down with ice and a little stir of the straw and I do exactly the same if I have a small glass of a fizzy soft drink.

Hair

You will hear so many things about how to protect your hair. Lotions and potions and drinks to help to prevent it from falling out, different ways how to help regrowth etc. The latest I heard this week was to rub rosemary oil into your scalp. Let's think about this for a minute. Apart from ending up smelling like a bit of roast lamb, if this actually worked we would all be doing it and I could sell the sprigs from my rosemary bush for £1000 each. The cold hard truth is that you can expect to have some hair loss, and for each individual person, the volume of hair loss is different. For me, I didn't lose lots of hair rapidly, it happened as a gradual process and as quickly as it came out, new hair began to grow, at times I looked like I had lots of sprouts of baby hair, which I guess I did. Some people say to take biotin and collagen before your op and continue taking it, some people say don't bother. Some say it helped, others say it hasn't. At the end of the day, your body will go through a huge shock which can cause hair loss and your body is receiving fewer nutrients which can also contribute towards hair loss.

I had hair extensions put in around eight months post-surgery, however when they came out, I had even less hair left. Then I had this crazy sprout of growth with lots of new hair. I have kept my hair fairly short, going back and forth from a long bob to a pixie cut. That is a style choice rather than needing to. There are plenty of people with long hair who have had weight loss surgery and maintained their long hair. I feel it helps my hair when I take biotin and collagen along with my multivitamins. My hair feels much thicker and stronger when I am taking those.

I have also used topical products such as caffeine shampoo, had my hair lightened through toner rather than bleach and used a detox shampoo so that it doesn't get heavy with products. I still do these things today. I have swapped to using **Silk Pillowcases** to help limit hair breakage when asleep. During my research, I read how these pillowcases can support your hair due to your hair not rubbing on a normal pillowcase overnight. Do I think it has helped? Yes,

I do. My hair is certainly less "rubbed" when using one when I wake up.

Hair loss is an issue for many people who have gastric surgery. There are gastric surgery patients who do lose a lot of hair and they do go on to wear wigs for a period of time whilst their body settles and becomes used to its new life. If that happens to you, try not to worry, as distressing as it may be. If you want to wear a wig, seek a great wig maker and use it to your advantage.

A friend of mine had a gastric bypass and almost all of her super curly hair slowly fell away. She said she had prepared as she had been advised it might happen. She went wig shopping and bought three different wigs. One for the week, one for the weekend and one for special occasions. It was incredible and she looked amazing. Once her hair had regrown - and was certainly full enough to not wear a wig - she continued to wear them on and off, simply for a change. And why not? There is always a solution to every problem. You just have to seek the right solution to suit yourself.

Energy

It is interesting when I have spoken to people who are dieticians or other medical people who haven't had surgery, as their immediate comment is often, along the lines of *"you may feel you have less energy each day"* or *"do you have less energy now you eat less"* and my answer is always, *"no"*. My energy is higher than it has ever been, and my determination to better myself in all avenues is also sky-high. As mentioned earlier, unless I stop looking after myself which causes a dip, my energy is great.

I would say that from the moment I started the LRD, I began to gain energy, not lose it. Personally, I think it is because I now don't eat all the rubbish and quick-fix sugar kicks that I used to eat, which would see my energy peak for a short period and then slump again, sometimes even lower than it did before. I can remember being around my heaviest weight and actually taking an afternoon nap before the school run because I was so fatigued.

There may be times when your energy naturally diminishes, or maybe you forget to eat, yes that is an actual thing as you just won't feel hungry. Amazing, right, that you may now forget to eat? Due to this, your energy may dip which will make you realise you need to have something to eat. Your body will talk to you, listen to it.

Apart from that, or the fact you may have been to a gym class and run there and back (no, I haven't achieved that just yet) then your energy should be of a great level. So don't listen to the naysayers on this one, because it simply isn't true. If you are regularly feeling fatigued post-surgery, please get a full checkup from your medical team. It isn't normal.

Sugar

One thing I do find that I do is, rather than check fat and calories, I check the sugar content. I find this limits any chance of sugar dumping and opens me up to many more foods that I would have previously discounted. One of these would be peanut butter. I didn't know until I began really looking into the foods that worked well for me, that peanut butter - the natural version - is full of health-promoting nutrients like magnesium, iron, vitamin E and vitamin B6. It has a good mix of protein and carbohydrates and is really nice when you feel like you want something to give you a sweet fix, without being full of refined sugar.

Back up

I do try and keep a nutritional shake powder in the house that I can mix with milk should I find that I am either running late and don't have anything I can grab and eat with ease, or if I am having a busy day and don't get the opportunity to either sort food, e.g., lunch for work, or if I know that where I am going will only have limited food options such as a jacket spud or sandwich. I don't rely on it, but it is a handy backup.

That is key for us, that we always have a handy backup so we don't revert to old habits that won't contribute to our success.

Forcefields up.
Manage yourself
to maintain your
success

X

11

TRANSFER ADDICTION

The first time I heard about transfer addiction, I dismissed it. *"I am not addicted to anything,"* I thought, therefore I have no addiction that will transfer. However, it is a real thing and certainly something for you to be aware of. Looking back, I was addicted to emotional eating and chocolate, and most likely still am, but, due to my gastric sleeve and working on my mindset with the tools we have discussed, that is in check.

People do struggle with transfer addiction. An example would be people who have come off of alcohol or drugs and have become uber marathon runners, their addiction transferred to extreme exercise.

There are gastric surgery patients who are post-surgery and have become addicted to exercise, sex, alcohol, or cleaning, for example. It is a real issue and something I felt was only right to make you aware of. So stick it on your radar and be aware of your choices. Obviously, don't overly worry if it is a benefit like cleaning - you could come and do mine if you need to get more of your fix. I will wholeheartedly support you.

If I had to say that something increased or transferred as I lost weight, it would be self-development. It started with listening to podcasts and audiobooks as I kept myself busy and it continued from there. I found that I wanted to improve and develop and help others. It is how I founded and created Gastric Surgery: The Lived Experience. The whole surgery process has hugely changed my life and now that of others.

This may make you sit upright and take note, interestingly, my sex drive rapidly went through the roof. Hold on, what was that? Did you just read that bit again? Haha. Yep, you read it again and you were correct the first time. As I lost weight, my sex drive went up and up and up. More on that later... off you go, flicking through the pages to find the bit on sex drive.....

Unpeeling the layers
day by day
for your new life,
your way

x

12

HOW YOU FEEL AS YOU LOSE WEIGHT

Losing weight through gastric surgery is almost indescribable. It is sort of effortless. Don't get me wrong, you will put the effort in, just in other ways. Gone are the days of the traditional dieting that you may have tried, where a 2lb loss was a real win. Now, you simply focus on eating small, drinking well to stay hydrated, and following some basic and simple rules and the weight, well the weight basically melts off. It can actually be oddly shocking. I used to think, "*absolutely no way have I lost 98lb*" as I was still losing weight, or there would be times when I was in the changing rooms and would have to take all of the size 20, then size 18, then size 16, then size 14, the size 12 clothes back and reach for a size 10, shaking my head in disbelief as I headed back to the changing rooms. I would stand in front of the mirror thinking *"is this really me?"* *"Ha! This IS really me"*.

There are times that you will feel incredible, and then there are times when you will be thinking what have I done? Mix a bit of body dysmorphia in with that thought and for a moment in your day, or sometimes for a whole day, you won't actually be able to truly see how amazingly well you are doing. This is where you have to make sure you don't sabotage yourself, so focus on staying mentally strong, and focus on your next success be that more weight loss, keeping yourself nutritionally well, or revamping your wardrobe.

Be prepared for there to be times when you are shocked by your own transformation. Everything shrinks. For me, that feeling pretty much began around my first three-stone loss. I was walking my children to school before heading off to work and my shoe kept slipping off my foot. I was thinking *"What on Earth is going on? I just need to get them into school"*. I had to go home and change my shoes before heading in to work. The penny didn't even drop that my feet had lost weight at that point. Then I spent the whole day at work holding up my trousers. I went home and stood in front of the mirror and realised I looked like I was wearing trousers two sizes too big, and it turned out, I was.

As you lose weight there will be even more unexpected things that will happen which no one made me aware of.

Back around the six to nine months post-op point, I booked an emergency appointment with my GP. I had found a lump and I needed it to be checked. No, not in my boob, or my armpit or groin, but in my lower back, and I was really worried about what it could be. I went in and explained that it was hard, uncomfortable and painful at times. It ached and made it difficult for me to sit for long. My GP asked me to stand up and gently touched where it was, "*YES! It's there, that's it*" I said. And she laughed. I turned around and looked at her and being really worried I asked, "*oh no, what is it?*" and she said, "*Louise, that is nothing to worry about, you have lost so much weight you have found your coccyx*". Well, blow me down. I don't think I have felt my coccyx for years. I am an astute person, however, at this moment in time, felt like a right wally. We then had a chat about how I was doing and for the first time, in as many years as I could remember, I was classed as a healthy weight. Sure, my BMI could still be lower, however at 5ft, to have what our national health considers a good BMI I have to weigh around the same weight as an ant's testicle. She was happy with my results and I was over the moon that a) she was happy and b) I had a coccyx.

If you are post-surgery, what have been the things that have taken you by surprise?

As you lose weight, you will rediscover your cheekbones, knees, elbows, ankles, collarbone and shoulder blades. They are actual bones in your body that, at some point, as we were gaining weight, we forgot ALL about. Believe me, they make a comeback. A bit like your favourite childhood singer, they manage to make a massive comeback. You begin to realise when you can't get comfortable in bed because your knees are knocking together, what feels like, bone on bone. That is where the pillow you used post-surgery, the duvet, or your partner's legs, become invaluable to pop between your knees so they don't rub together and you can get to sleep. #usefulpartner

WHAT HAPPENS?

Your clothes and hairstyle will no doubt change in some way as you begin to change body shape. Not necessarily completely, however, you will become more refreshed and be willing to try new shapes and styles. I absolutely love wearing jumpsuits and dresses now, whereas beforehand, I was always reluctant, or if I did I spent the whole time awfully self-conscious. I love wearing colourful clothes now. If I find something that I like now, I will often buy it in a couple of colours. There are some well-known shops and brands that I have found I really love that suit my shape and new style. I have always loved people who can get things to match like bags and shoes and I was never able to get that to happen very well. Now, I can, I love it. The other thing that is a bit weird is that we can now shop in shops that are almost extremes, like much cheaper or much more expensive AND we can make the clothes from the cheaper shops look more expensive as they fit us better. That's a win-win in my book.

I have a newfound love of wearing heels, why? Because they now fit my feet nicely and it doesn't kill my knees any more. My clothes selection has become more colourful and there are so many more shops available to shop in too. I have realised that the shop sizes do not actually match each other. What could be a size 10 in one shop could be a 14 in another. That was a revelation because some shops make you feel like you are bigger than you are, so watch out for those sneaky so and so's.

There will be times when you just don't know what to wear or how to dress because your body is so different and you have so many options. Try it all on and see what new style your new body takes you to. And your style may change regularly, I don't think I have found one particular style as I like quite a few now.

It is like we are all like Russian dolls, where you peel back one layer and find the next small doll inside. Or like a human pass-the-parcel. As each layer comes off, we find a nice surprise, like collarbones. Each 7lbs feels as if the next layer has been unwrapped.

Do keep hold of an item or two of clothes that you had as you went into surgery. The rest, feel free to donate to charity or sell on. As you lose weight, keep trying on your old item of clothing. You will be amazed at how it feels. I can remember getting both of my legs into one of the legs of my old jeans, and I now have a photo of me in my son's jeans, who was 12 years old at the time, so keep one item, it really is enlightening. Especially if you have a day where you cant see your progress any more, it will help remind you how far you have come.

RIB ACHE

I honestly do not think anyone would expect to have this. I experienced aching ribs from around the three-stone weight loss point. You may not experience it at all, but then again, you might. Just like with a lot of the symptoms and things we will personally experience, it is personal to you. I have seen and had many people ask about this so feel it is something to highlight to you.

I began to develop an ache around my rib cage and if I am honest, I was really worried. I was six to eight weeks post-surgery and my weight loss was going really well. So I called the surgical team at the hospital as all sorts of questions were running through my head - maybe I was bleeding inside? Maybe I had an internal leak? I was totally fearing the worst... Oh, how wrong could I be?

I made the call and explained my situation, going into as much detail as I could regarding achy ribs. I explained that I was achy, all around my rib cage and answered their questions. Yes, it was at the front as well as the back and yes, around the sides. No, I didn't have any temperature. No, I wasn't sweating. No, I didn't feel sick. No, I wasn't pale.

I was thinking, am I supposed to be worried? Is there something seriously wrong? The questions continued. Yes, I could eat. Yes, I could drink. Yes, I could bend. *"Well Louise, we have to tell you that your rib cage is shrinking"*. I stood for a moment on the end of the phone and thought *"What? Shrinking?"* I said. *"Hold on a minute, I'm not tall enough as it is, I can't be shrinking"*. *"No"*, the nurse laughed. *"YOU are not shrinking, although you probably are with your weight loss. Your rib cage is slowly pulling in as it adjusts to your surgery and also the fact that you are losing weight. It is actually quite common"*, the nurse said, *"it's just not that well known"*. Well, knock me down with a feather, Trevor! My ribs are aching because they are pulling in as my body gets smaller. And I laughed. I said I couldn't believe that was an actual thing and she said, *"Well, it sure is and it means you are doing really well"*. So I thanked her for the reassurance and my goodbyes.

I would have NEVER thought you could get achy ribs from losing weight, but I can confirm that you can. I went and bought myself a soft corset to wear to support my ribs which did help. The ache didn't last for too long, it would start and last around a week or so and then would go and then, every now and then, come back again.

Then there are the times that you may get picked up. I don't mean by a curb crawler, or by someone thinking they have got lucky on a night out, I mean physically picked up. It is the last thing that I a) expected to happen and b) quite liked happening.

The first time it happened I was on a night out with some friends and some guys were out dressed as firefighters. Actually looking back, they may well have been actual firefighters. However, either way, there was a group of them outside the bar we had been to. As we walked by, one of the girls said something and the next thing I know I was being lifted in the air as if they were lifting a toddler! I was so shocked and was laughing, saying put me down, and I'm too heavy. The guy said to me, you aren't heavy as he began to run up and down the street with me.

The second time it happened, I was on a date with my now husband and we were dancing at a music gig and he said to get on his shoulders, I said absolutely no way, not a chance. So he picked me up! I know he would have known how I was feeling. Nervous, excited, scared, shocked, and happy, so he picks me up from time to time now, which I think is his way of reminding me how light I am compared to before.

Then there are the armpits that change shape. Whether you are male or female, they suddenly become hollow and shaving and putting deodorant on needs a whole new skill set. Although shaving does become quicker as there is less of you to shave.

There are the weird things you will suddenly be able to do, like hold your own hands behind your back, see your feet easily, run for a bus or after a child without even thinking about it. You may bounce on a trampoline for fun without fear of judgement. Find courage or dig out the "who cares" attitude like I did and pop a bikini on whether you are in the garden or at the beach and enjoy the sun and the breeze on your skin, which you may not have done in a very long time. The list is endless and the moments of joy are endless too.

Oh, the journey of weight loss surgery and of losing weight!

Managing every

situation becomes

a breeze

X

13

EATING OUT

Eating out is something that you will do, and you will slowly be able to work your own way to navigate the restaurant landscape.

When I had my surgery, if you asked for a small portion, tried to order off of the kid's menu or have a starter as a main, everyone looked at you as if you had grown three heads and clearly you must have some sort of eating disorder. If you asked for a box to take the food home in, you were either told no, due to reheating concerns (I will never forget that comment, it was a chicken salad), or you were visually assessed for being really financially tight. Thankfully, now, pretty much anything goes and taking food out or having a starter as a main isn't looked upon as weird.

I really enjoy eating out. I enjoy going out more than I ever have before and I feel this is most likely because I feel good, mentally and physically. I am really happy to be able to share with you the way I have learnt to navigate eating out and hope that it will bring you some ideas and also some reassurance and comfort that there are many of us out there that don't eat large main meals.

I have a couple of rules that I follow to ensure I can enjoy the food I eat and the time out with whoever I am with.

- I order food that isn't too dry or if it is a sandwich, it has to have a filling that isn't overly dry. Bread needs moisture otherwise it turns into a plug.
- I order something from the starter menu if I can and if I don't fancy anything, I order something that I can box up and take home from the main menu.
- I aim to order a dish or dishes that are high in protein.
- I try to stay away from bread or heavy-carb dishes.

So that I don't get myself into a situation where food gets stuck, more than ever I stick to the 20-20-20 rule.

I am also fortunate that if I am eating out with people who are aware of my surgery, I share a couple of starters and a main meal with them as a sharing platter type dinner, like a tapas, I suppose. When I say *"people"*, I heavily encourage my husband to share his main meal with me with added sides. I can't say he is always over-enamoured with this as he loves his own food, but he does do it to support me.

Speaking of tapas, for me, that is one of the easiest restaurants to go to eat at. We have a Spanish tapas near us, an Indian restaurant who do curry tapas, smaller dishes of a wider selection of curry and an Italian that do a selection of smaller plates. And there are now lots of menus which have smaller dishes on, which are really handy for all of us who have had surgery. I am sure you will have your favourites or go to places that you have found or will find that are great for you.

I enjoy all restaurants and I am no saint. I have a sweet tooth and would happily forgo all other foods and head straight to the dessert section if I could, however, that isn't why I had my surgery, and potentially that sweet tooth goes some way as to why I have had surgery. I try to maintain my mindset to focus on nutritional consumption rather than just sugar and risk a sugar dump.

Some restaurants are absolutely terrible for us to eat in - the ones where they serve processed, carbohydrate-heavy meals with no or minimal salad or nutritious protein options. Those ones, I will avoid if I can. I point-blank refuse to give them my custom. Then there are those who trade as carbohydrate-heavy, however, they actually have other meals that are high in protein and other nutrition. I'm thinking of one well-known pizza restaurant and its sister Italian restaurant - now they do have some great meals we can choose from like protein pasta and protein salad and side dishes. The key thing is to do some research beforehand if you can and if you can't, make the best of the situation you find yourself in.

I have had lunches and dinners out with friends or with work, and have had to be creative on what I do and don't order. I have found that menus often have high protein salads on, so if they do, I will order one, eat the protein and then once I am full, will leave the remaining salad along with a comment like *"gosh, I can't eat all those leaves"*. Weirdly, people normally agree, as if eating leaves is filling so it is acceptable to leave them. I bet if I left half a pizza someone would want a piece. Guaranteed.

If you attend events such as festivals, there is often a jacket potato van, which can be handy. Although the potato is not high in protein itself, the toppings often are like baked beans, cheese, chilli con carne and tuna, all of which can also be easy to eat and digest for us.

Here's an example of the way I managed my lunch choice this week. I went to see a client and we had lunch at a hotel bar. I ordered a chicken and avocado mayo sandwich and they ordered a cheese and ham sandwich, the sandwich was heavily carb loaded. When they arrived, I cut off the crusts and removed one layer of the bread and ate it as an open sandwich. My client did the same and added the side salad onto the top of her sandwich. We both enjoyed them and we ate until we were full. There are plenty of ways and means that you can manage the foods you have when you are eating out to suit you.

I have also found that I really like more vegetarian and vegan dishes than I would have thought. I enjoy the high-protein lentils and pulses along with the vegetables and cheeses these different dishes often offer.

With so much time
available,
your future could
be brighter in
so many ways

X

14

THE HABIT OF HUNGER

I am sure you have heard that saying before, the habit of hunger. Head hunger or eye hunger, over actual body hunger, often takes the lead.

Now that your hunger hormone has been removed from your stomach, or has at least been greatly reduced, hunger can only really be a habit. I bet you have a favourite cupboard you just can't help but open when you go into the kitchen. Or a habit that, you know, makes you look inside the fridge, just because you are near the fridge. Perhaps you have a habit of coffee and cake on Thursday because you know, it's nearly the weekend, or Friday night takeaway, Saturday evening movie and popcorn night and ice cream on Sundays after Sunday lunch. Then there is the McDonalds on the way home from swimming, *"No kids, I'm not having one, I will eat with your Dad*" or your own version of this answer, as you swallow a kid's cheeseburger on the drive home. I know the story, I know the drill, I have lived it. I am sometimes surprised I didn't wear the hinges off of my 'cupboard' and fridge.

One night, after a long day of being at work, doing the washing, popping the hoover round and finally sorting dinner, I was feeling really 'meh'. The hunger habit saw its opportunity and kicked in. I was a single mum at the time and because the children were in bed, I couldn't go for a walk around the block, gardening wasn't going to fix this craving, and in the end, I actually found myself standing in the kitchen chewing through a packet of the kids pack lunch crisps. Rather than swallowing the crisps, I was standing over the bin and spitting them out. Looking back, how utterly ridiculous. I have absolutely no idea what I was doing, although, at that moment in time, it seemed to make complete sense. Would I recommend it to you? Absolutely not, as it makes you look like a complete weirdo and it wastes food. At the time it served a purpose, and I'm quite proud that I spat them out rather than swallow them as slider food so I guess it served a purpose and I achieved some sort of a small win.

You see, we eat and drink out of habit. It is comforting, it is the usual for us and we recognise happiness or fulfilment in eating. We perhaps eat more or the wrong things when we are tired, we make up for lost time by eating to catch up for the times we were dieting. Crazy, right? But it's true. I bet one of you has left a slimming club and picked up a takeaway or at least ordered it for delivery on the way home because, you know, it's weigh day and you have been weighed and it's still the same day so won't affect tomorrow. I've done it myself.

Now that you have your new stomach, and you have been through a lot of the hard work, what can you do to ensure that you introduce new habits to replace the old ones? Preparing my kitchen cupboards before surgery really helped. I'm an awful snacker and I have had to work really hard to make sure snacking hasn't sabotaged my weight loss. One of the things that I have done is to make sure that I have high protein or highly nutritious things to snack on when I fancy snacking e.g. when I am not able to full control the head craving. In the fridge, I have things like Babybel, chopped chicken, raspberries and blueberries, sliced meats, boiled eggs, frittata and soups. I also have things like hot milk lattes, protein balls and protein bars. They are the things that help me from snacking on the wrong things, they protect my weight loss and any further sabotage when I just can't seem to fully break the habit.

Sometimes it is because I am cold and that is when the hot milk lattes and soup helps.

When I realised that I still had the habit of going to '**the**' cupboard even after I cleared most of the cupboards out pre-surgery, I decided that it was time to change the cupboards around, so the cupboard that used to contain all of the stuff that I would snack on which was no good for me, now contained pots and pans. Changing your habits is literally you changing the pathways in your brain from what you used to do, to what you now need to do, re-writing your neurological pathways. There have been times when I would have still emotionally eaten and have actually taken myself into the garden and done some gardening, had a bath or walked around the block to try and control or change my mindset, to change my habits. Your mindset change isn't going to happen overnight and it is something that you have to work on to make sure you achieve long-term success. You absolutely can do it, I truly believe you can and am a living success that it is possible to take back control. You may have to have a rest every now and again, however, you can gain control.

I did form my own tactics to get the head hunger in check. My daughter was seven when I had my surgery. She loves to sing and dance. One of the tactics I used was to get her to put on one of her favourite song tracks and we would sing and dance along. All I needed was 10 minutes or so to reset my mind and I would make sure I would have a drink at the same time, to trick my mind that I had had something. We would sing and dance along to all sorts of soundtracks and as she has got older, now 14, I have to say it is something we still do if one of us has had a rough day, or we just want to have a good laugh. Kitchen and car karaoke are firm favourites.

My son was nine when I had my surgery. He loves sports, and gaming, however, as a single mum with a son who loves sports, I am sure those of you who are in the same situation know that you have to try and be a dad as well as a mum at times. I would offer him a game of footie or ball throwing in the garden. In the spring and summer, we would spend ages out in the garden playing games and chatting, and occasionally the 'annoying' younger sister would come and join in, although she is competitive so would give him a run for his money way more than I could. As it turns out, I am a dab hand at badminton with the camping set I bought from a well-known, lower-priced supermarket chain. Who would have thought I could whip my children at a game of badminton, definitely not pre-surgery.

I would also clean. Mainly in the evenings, when the boredom head hunger would set in. I decided that rather than try and fight the head hunger by sitting, I would do a job whilst having a warm drink to occupy my mind. I was really proud of myself that I managed to sort through lots of cupboards, wardrobes and paperwork that I had left to do *"later"*. I'm not sure my husband would agree with that now as I have refilled wardrobes with new clothes and shoes, however, I did do it. I promise I did.

You may undertake a new course to study, re-write your CV and look for a new job or a change of career direction. The world is your oyster. Use your time to your advantage. I took some courses and studied and I also began to coach other patients in readiness for their surgery. There is so much you can do, try something new or do that one thing you have always wanted to do yet always put off.

At the end of the day, you have to do things that work for you in each given situation. If it's towards you maintaining or achieving further weight loss, that's all that matters. Spend 10 minutes scrubbing the loo if it stops you from reaching for slider foods. I believe in you, you have got this.

It is most

definitely NOT

all a

load of shit

x

15

LET'S TALK POO

Haha. I bet you weren't expecting this chapter.

Poo is something that you are going to spend a bit of time thinking about, possibly even talking about and you are certainly going to spend a bit of time trying to do. Let's look at this logically for a minute, the less you put in, the less is going to come out. That is the fact of the matter.

I am no dietician, and I am no digestive expert, however, over the last 6+ years I have become an expert on having a poo: What I need to eat to ensure that I do poo, how to manage constipation and how to do my best to not become constipated. Delightful topic, 100% necessary.

In a conversation with a friend, who I must point out is a nurse, I explained how I was really struggling to go to the toilet and had done so for some time. It would give me headaches, make me feel pretty rubbish in my tummy and it would really hurt when I did manage to go, which, due to how long it took, meant I had put a stack of books in the loo to read. She said to me, "*Louise, you need more fibre in your diet, in any shape or form that you can eat*" and explained how not going regularly really isn't great for your bowel in the long run.

It can be really tricky if you don't manage yourself and regulate things properly to support your bowel. I do think that due to our style of diet, and the fact that our food intake is a lot smaller, it means that we poo less, I mean we must do, right? But, we can certainly do the best we can in supporting our bodies to ensure we do actually poo, and poo regularly to help keep our bowels healthy.

I spent some time looking at high-fibre foods and trying things out to see what would work for me. Here is an example of high-fibre foods and other things that I mix through my weekly food and drink to support my bowel movement:

- Popcorn - A basic salted, small bag works a treat.
- A vegetable soup.
- Baked beans - high in protein too.
- Keeping on top of water intake.

- A daily probiotic.
- Porridge. Which is a complex carbohydrate and provides fibre.
- Lentils mixed through homemade dinners and salads.
- Mixed plain nuts.
- Vegetables and some fruits such as apples.

All of those things help me to maintain my bowel movement and poo, so hopefully, they will also be useful to you too.

Make a list here of the foods you have eaten this week and check to see if they are high in fibre. It will really help you to understand how much you are having and where you may need to increase your fibre intake.

Food	How much fibre per 100g

Be brilliant.

Ensure you achieve

all that you can

x

16

SELF-EFFICACY AND RESILIENCE

The first time I heard the word self-efficacy was on a podcast and the story made me really sit up and listen, to the point that I played it four times. The person being interviewed was explaining how people with high self-efficacy do better than those who have lower self-efficacy or who do not strive to have higher self-efficacy. He spoke about people who have come from or fallen into very tricky situations, or situations that they didn't want to be in and through their own self-efficacy, they made positive and sustained changes to their life.

Self-efficacy is a person's belief in their ability to complete a task or achieve a goal, the drive to achieve what they want to achieve, and having the strong, positive belief that they have the capacity and the skills to achieve their goals.

Self-efficacy is the belief that we can achieve positive influences over the conditions that affect our lives and exert a positive influence over our own environment. Self-efficacy encompasses a person's confidence in themselves to control their own behaviour and stay motivated in the pursuit of their own goal.

People can have self-efficacy in different situations and places, such as at home, school, work, in all relationships, and in all other areas important to themselves. Oddly, since hearing this and looking into it, I feel that my own self-efficacy has helped all areas of my life.

It helps me to understand that I am solely responsible for what I eat and drink, and self-efficacy helps me to achieve my weight loss goals and sustained weight loss. Self-efficacy helps me to keep getting up, getting out of bed and heading for a walk, going for a swim or heading to the gym. Self-efficacy has helped me when I have struggled with food and drinks post-operation, and in making the right choices for the benefit of my body and overall life.

Self-efficacy has helped me when body dysmorphia has kicked in when I have looked in the mirror and only seen the old Louise. It kicked my butt to the curb and made me see the new Louise, the actual Louise standing in front of the mirror.

Self-efficacy makes me realise that actually, this is all on me. Everything I am doing is my choice, my choices are my own and I always have a choice - even if that is to eat nothing at that moment and wait until later for a better option rather than spit the crisps out in the bin. I always have a choice.

Self-efficacy goes hand in hand nicely with resilience and we need a fair amount of that too. As people who have been overweight and have decided to do something about it for the long term, we already have fairly high resilience, we just need to use it to our advantage, post-surgery. Add in some self-efficacy, and we are all individual successful forces to be reckoned with.

It has been my self-efficacy that has picked me back up when I have almost derailed. It has been my self-efficacy that kept me focused when I was on my LRD. It has been my self-efficacy that has supported my mind and body to maintain my weight loss and if any lbs start to creep back on, it nudges me back on track.

Self-efficacy more than likely was part of the process of deciding to have surgery and make a strong change. Without believing that I was able to have surgery and be successful, I don't feel I would have been as successful as I am today.

You will all have some level of self-efficacy, take some time to consider how high yours is and what you can do to raise your level so that you continually move forward and achieve great things, not just with your weight, but in all areas of your life.

Hey sexy,

I'm home

X

17

SEX DRIVE - KABOOM

Now, I don't think it is just me, but did you know that when you lose weight your sex drive goes up? No? You didn't know that? To be honest, neither did I. I heard it somewhere and to this day I'm not sure if it is due to the hormones that are released with the loss of the extra weight we are carrying, or if we just feel amazing, however, my sex drive rapidly increased. Perhaps it could be due to losing weight and feeling better mentally and physically or maybe there is some actual science behind it. As I lost weight, my sex drive increased like you wouldn't believe and when I met the man that is now my husband, let's just say, we partook in a lot of extracurricular activities. Lucky man.

Referring back to transfer addiction, the drive to want to feel good and have great sex far outweighs the addiction to food, which also supports our new lives. Depending on where you are in your journey, think about what has happened for you, and if the rise in sex drive has kicked in. Tag me with a #Kaboom on my Instagram, Gastric Surgery: The Lived Experience if it has and don't you dare all come back to me and say you are pregnant. I will not be held accountable for increasing the world population.

The nice thing is if sexy undies are your thing - or your partner's - well, hello sailor, now is the time to get them out or buy some new ones. You may be able to try new positions and enjoy all of the new feels this brings with it. Enjoy anything and everything that you may have been missing out on.

I have no complaints and neither does my husband. I wonder if there is actually any correlation between gastric surgery and a rise in pregnancy rates...

Baby,
it's not actually
cold outside

X

18

FEELING THE COLD

It makes me feel cold just by typing the word cold. I wish someone had told me that we will feel the cold a lot more than we did before. I am currently sitting writing this book with my feet in an electric foot warmer and have a vest on under my top. Not a word of a lie.

Some people have said to me it is because I have lost the "*padding*" from losing weight - cheeky sods - and maybe that is true, but still, they don't need to say it right.

Some people say it is because my metabolism has slowed down due to the rapid weight loss through gastric surgery and maybe that is true, though I don't think it is. Some people have said that I am low in iron, and maybe that is true, although my blood checks all come back healthy and normal, so I don't think that is the case.

Whatever it may be, I feel the cold. Do you? I love being warm and will happily sit in the sun like a cat getting the nice warmth on my face and body. Especially in the winter.

There are plenty of ways to help you keep warm. The colder I get, the more I want to eat or snack on, so keeping warm is key for me. Some of the things I do to keep warm and not look like an Eskimo even mid-summer are:

- Wear a vest under my tops
- Use an electric foot warmer or a hot water bottle on my feet
- Walk or do some exercise first thing in the morning, this helps to get my body going and raise my overall body temperature
- Have regular warm drinks
- Use blankets on the sofa and on top of the duvet
- I take a large scarf with me everywhere.

I have bought a car with a heated seat and steering wheel and I am not ashamed to use them in the summer as well as the winter. I will sit right next to, on top of if I can, the warmest person in the house, which is my husband. He is defo the warmest person around - he radiates heat and I am sure he thinks that I really love him which is why I cuddle in, I do love him, but if only he knew the deeper truth...

Honey,

I shrunk.....

myself

X

19

SHRINKING IN SIZE AND
BECOMING YOU

W hen you begin to lose weight, you are shrinking. You suddenly start to shrink rapidly, and in areas, you may not have even thought of. As I mentioned earlier, effectively, everything on me has shrunk, my feet, hands, waist, chest, back, bottom, legs, face... you name it, I reckon it has shrunk.

My feet have gone from a size 5.5 to a 4.5. My hands are thinner, I have gone down four ring sizes and I have had to get the rings I want to wear resized. My wrists shrunk and my watch actually bruised my new boney wrist. Your hands and wrist sort of happen without you realising. In fact, it all sort of happens without you realising things are changing.

The clothes I buy have gone down from a size 20-22 to a size 10-12. At my smallest, I even wore a few things that were a size 8. It does depend on where you shop and on your shape so please do not compare yourself to anyone else. I am giving you these as a rough guide as I personally share my journey with you. Today at 6 years and 8 months post-op, I ordered a pair of size 12 jeans and they fit lovely. I am a happy lady.

I shrunk in size so much that you could actually see my breastbone. And you know what, that wasn't quite where I wanted to be as I had also lost my breasts. I had gone from a 40 EE cup to a 34 C cup and things didn't feel quite right. For me, the seven-stone loss was too low.

I had the issue where I now realised I had a coccyx, and that would regularly get in my way as my bottom had shrunk. I had painful bones where they would knock or catch on things, like my wrist bones on the desk at work or my ankles inside my boots. Don't get me wrong, I was amazed that I had lost seven stones, however, I wasn't quite happy with my loss.

Although I had lost weight and had been walking, I hadn't done any proper exercise to build up muscle tone, so I began first with classes I knew I would enjoy, like aquafit and Zumba, and then began to do some weight training. I don't do lots of strength and conditioning, so when I do, it is hard work... and yes, after the delayed onset muscle soreness, which you will hear gym bunnies refer to as DOMS, has worn off, I always feel great.

I have a friend who regularly weight trains and at 5ft 2in can deadlift 90kg. I think that is quite a lot for someone of her size and I am impressed. I know building muscle builds metabolism, which supports weight loss, so if this does become your thing, don't forget you will begin to weigh more, despite feeling and measuring smaller, as your body shape changes as you build muscle.

So I did some exercise to build muscle tone and I also put on 7 lbs, slowly and carefully and I now mentally feel and physically feel that I look right.

DATING AND RELATIONSHIPS

Four months after my operation, my marriage broke down. Did I see it coming? Yes, I did. Perhaps it was all part of the new me and the new life, however, we had already grown apart quite a while before my operation. After almost exactly two years to the day post-surgery, I met the man who is now my husband. Although I had been on a couple of dates, he was the first man I properly dated and spoke to about my surgery.

I decided that

a) he didn't need to know it all at once,

and

b) I needed to know that I could trust him before I told him everything.

The reason I made this decision is that I had opened up to some people who I believed were close friends whom I could trust and they immediately judged me and my decision. They made assumptions and accusations without even asking me the full details of why I had chosen to have gastric surgery, which was a real shame. Some people said, well they weren't your actual friends, and maybe they weren't, however at the time, and certainly for the years before, I believed that they were and as our relationships broke down, for me, and possibly for them, it was a tricky time to navigate.

I had had two years of getting to know the new me so I was secure in my new body and lifestyle. We were having a great time together, I knew l really liked him, therefore it was key to me that I took things as carefully as I introduced my surgery to him so I didn't get hurt.

The first time we went out for food, I joked and said to him, so that you know, I will be the cheapest or the most expensive date you will ever have. He looked at me and I said, well I will either only order a starter or I will order a fillet steak (I can eat fillet steak really well, no idea why I just can, my sleeved stomach seems to love it) he laughed thinking I was joking. I said I'm not joking, you will see. The first meal I ever had with him was a ribbon courgette and scallop starter. On the second date, I had fillet steak. I broke him in gently.

It took me about three months before I told him any more of the details. I began by first saying that I had had a stomach operation and therefore my stomach was reduced. He said, *"cool"*, that was it, and we began talking about our children. About a month later, I said, you know I said I have a smaller stomach due to an operation, well, it is because I chose to have ¾ of my stomach removed. He said, *"cool"*, and that was pretty much that. He has never asked about the operation itself in detail. He has asked things like, what foods are easier for me to eat and what types of food do I need to eat, and when he is looking for restaurants, he will point-blank refuse to go to those that have a starter menu full of bread and beige.

Looking back, he literally didn't care at all. Not one bit. And he still doesn't. I know that he is my main cheerleader and will always defend me to the hilt. There is something very refreshing in that and I really hope you have your own cheerleader in some shape or form. If you don't, I will be yours.

If you find the right people, they don't care that you have had weight loss surgery, they just care that you are happy and successful. That is key for your own well-being and also your own success for your future.

There may be times when your resilience comes into play along with your self-efficacy, where people are not kind nor understanding and you have to say, you are just not my person, and walk away. What I can tell you is that your people are out there, either with you now or waiting to be found.

EXCESS SKIN

I don't overly suffer from excess skin. Sure, I would like my stomach to be tighter or flatter, but after two c-sections and weight loss surgery, it would have been a miracle if it had all suddenly pulled back in flat all by itself. Maybe my arms could be a bit more toned and perhaps the top of my legs to be tighter... crikey, wouldn't we all like something to be tighter or firmer, even people who haven't had weight loss surgery. I am sure body brushing helped, I really am. I also think the fact I walked lots and gently exercised with pilates fairly early on helped my muscles too.

You can use knickers to suit your shape and hold your stomach in, which can help when wearing a posh frock. It does me. I quite like the softer body corsets I wore when my ribs were achy. They support well under a dress too. There has been an odd time that my skin has been sore, and if this is something that you have experienced, then I really do send my love to you. I am fully aware that it will all be individual as it will depend on your own skin and your own individual weight loss.

With my arms, I have learnt not to worry about them, along with my legs. People can have their thoughts and I will have a nice time regardless. Before I became brave, I did wear capped sleeves and ¾ sleeves more often, and the first time I wore shorts I nearly had a panic attack. Yet after I had worn them once, it became easier and easier. Blinking hell, shorts. I didn't own a pair for years, but now I have four pairs.

PLASTIC SURGERY

Some people choose to have plastic surgery to remove excess skin or for other reasons like boob lifts and I admire those who do as at times they can be big operations. This isn't something that I have chosen to do and more than likely won't. I have occasionally had a tantrum and said things like *"I need a tummy tuck"*, or *"That's it, I'm going to book a boob job, and they can sort my arms out at the same time"* as if it is some magical quick fix. I am sure you may have felt like that.

Some of you will have had or will choose to have plastic surgery, and some of you will be like me and think that you also feel that your body has been through enough. Our decisions are all personal.

I mentally feel really good, I'm very happy with the weight loss I have achieved and gone on to maintain. I don't feel that I need to put my body through any more surgery. That is my own personal decision and yours will be yours.

If you choose to have plastic surgery, follow the same process described earlier in the book. Do your research on your surgeon and medical team before you make your decision and prepare your body as well as you can.

Interestingly, when I am at the gym or the beach or just out and about, especially in the summer or at Christmas dos when people have their arms out, I look at other women and men and think, *"You know what, I'm doing alright"*. If I compare myself to a lean 24-year-old then, of course, I'm nowhere nearly as tight and toned in comparison, and that's ok, as they haven't lived the life that I have. If I feel people are looking at me or making any sort of judgement,

I have trained myself to laugh, give them a wink and think, *"If they've got the time to look at my body and make a negative judgement on any area of me, then they've got far too much time on their hands and they can come and do my ironing with it".* I hate ironing.

Your excess skin is yours and any decisions you are considering aren't something I would advise on. It is personal to you and how you feel and only you can decide what to do about it. I have learnt to treat mine as my friend. I look after my skin and moisturise it well, use supportive knickers, and a good bra and go about my day without a care in the world. We often think it is worse than it is. Good-natured people would rather celebrate your weight loss with you than comment on any excess skin.

You may decide to have plastic surgery and have your excess skin reduced, if you do then awesome and well done for making the decision that suits you. If your excess skin is getting you down, yet you don't want to have any more surgery, approach it from a different angle. Thank it for always being there with you and take it on the journey of its life as it is all part of your new body.

SCARS AND STRETCH MARKS.

My surgery scars healed really well. I used bio-oil to help with this and my scars are really minimal. I do think it depends on the neatness of your surgeon, your particular skin and again, how well you look after yourself post-surgery. They are there though, and they don't tan as well as the rest of my skin. On holiday, a couple of years ago, I was chatting to another holidaymaker, who asked if I had had my gallstones removed as they had. I said no I hadn't. They said, oh your scars look similar to mine. I just said *"oh, yes,"* and left it at that. What I actually thought was *"Nice one. If I am ever asked why I have my scars and don't want to say anything, I could always say it is due to having my gallbladder removed."*

My stretch marks are fairly minimal considering my weight fluctuations and weight loss. Everyone has them in some shape or form. I do feel body brushing helped and I have moisturised with bio-oil from time to time. Mine don't worry me, especially since I heard someone referring to them as tiger stripes and I feel I have earnt mine. Since then, that is how I think of mine. I earned them, through the ups and the downs over the years and the surgery process.

So, have I had anything else done? Yes, I have had botox as I felt I could use a helping hand on my extremely expressive forehead. I swear people can tell what I am thinking just by the way that my forehead moves. I am also currently going through the process of having my teeth straightened with Invisalign. I feel my teeth have moved or that they are clearer to see now that my face is slimmer. I have had to wait six years to be in a position where I could have it done after paying for my surgery. Again, I did my research on both of the people I am using. No doubt there may be other things as I age and change that I may have, however, any more major surgery is not currently on my list.

Sometimes your body just has to take a little time out,

just a little

x

20

WEIGHT LOSS STALL

A weight loss stall can, and most likely will happen to all of us at different points in our weight loss journey. You will have periods of rapid weight loss and then periods where things slow down or you stall for a while. I was advised by my medical team that I could stall for anywhere between three weeks to three months particularly around six months after surgery. Thankfully that didn't happen, but that isn't to say I haven't had stalls. I have, and I do regularly see people stall around the six-month point, post-surgery.

On my journey, I had a couple of times here and there where my weight loss stalled, for around two weeks each time. This stall was usually at the same time as the following things happening and it may help you to be aware of them. Yours may happen for different reasons and it would be useful to keep a track of what is or isn't going on when your stalls happen so that you can kick-start things going in the right direction.

I have made a list of the things that happened around the same time as my stalls for you so you can see which ones may also relate to you.

- When I had shrunk again and I needed to wear smaller clothes as if the stall was my body having a break before losing weight again
- When I realised that I wasn't drinking enough fluid
- When I realised I wasn't eating regularly enough
- When walking had slipped off of my radar due to not prioritising it in my day
- When I may have had some foods that were not nutritious but I like them, e.g., reverting to old habits
- Monthly period cycle
- Not sticking to the 20-20-20 rule
- Not sticking to the 30-minute rule.

It was almost as if my body was protecting itself. By putting itself into a stall, my body was saying "*Oi, buddy, we have been through enough, sort yourself out. We still have some more work to do,"* or *"I am just having a rest before we go again".*

Now, remember, there is no actual rhyme or reason why we stall. Our bodies are magnificent things, and you may never find the answer or the link to why you stall. I do recommend you keep yourself aware of what is happening because if you are still wanting to lose weight, it will help.

All of our bodies are different and we will all lose weight at a different rates and at different times, and our final weights will all be different and specific to us.

Use the journal on the next page to document the dates you stall for and to see if there is a link or a common theme. Don't worry so much about what you weigh because just knowing what you weigh isn't going to restart your losing weight, but knowing what is causing you, consciously or subconsciously, to stall will enable you to address whatever it is and allow you to begin to lose weight again.

Don't forget, sometimes your body literally just needs a week or two to regroup and catch up with itself. Love yourself, nurture yourself, and you will get through your stall.

Happy,
grateful,
and
living your
best life

X

21

YOUR HAPPY WEIGHT

O ne rule I do have is that I will not get into a detailed conversation with anyone who is over-opinionated about how much I weigh or weighed. I don't mind sharing what I weigh if I need or want to, however, if someone is overly opinionated about my weight or my weight loss journey, I close the conversation down. It is my body, my life and my journey, as is yours. Please do not ever feel pressured into disclosing your personal business to anyone.

This is not the case with you beautiful people. I hope that sharing my journey of surgery and weight loss is helpful to you. Let's face it, anyone who is against gastric surgery is most likely not going to read this book, and if they do, well, good on them, they will have learnt so many things and hopefully, it will change their thought process towards gastric surgery.

On the day of my surgery, I weighed 16st and 8lbs. My lowest weight was 9st 2lb. Today, my happy weight sits around 10st 7lbs.

My end weight is a weight I not only feel happy at, it is a weight that I can easily maintain without overthinking things. Absolutely there are times when I may gain a few lbs here and there, however, when I utilise all of the tools I have at my disposal, and all of the things I have learnt on my weight loss journey, and mix in some activity, I know I can get back into my happy weight zone, and I have proven that I can maintain it for years, as I have done.

Don't let anyone tell you what you should or shouldn't weigh, it is personal to you. For my height, if I was in the healthy BMI range as I mentioned earlier, I would have to weigh the same as an ants testicle, and even at my lowest weight of 9st 2lbs, I felt like I only just scraped into the healthy BMI range. Which is when I lost my boobs and you could see my chest bones and my hair went really thin.

So during your journey, remember that whatever your end weight is, make sure it makes you happy. Because if you are happy, your weight will stabilise and you will be able to maintain it well.

SCALES

You will either love them or hate them. When I decided to have surgery, I made a promise to myself that I would only weigh myself every month, and if I broke that promise, it would be no more than every two weeks. Generally, I weigh monthly now. Don't get me wrong though, I have to fight the curiosity of the daily weighing battle.

We can become obsessed with a number on the scales - I think that is why I decided that I needed a happy weight zone.

As I lost weight, I would say that the inches lost and the weight loss didn't always tally together. I never measured my inches, however, I know sometimes I would feel fuller and wouldn't expect to have lost weight, yet would have lost lbs and then the next time would feel slimmer, thinking I had lost lots and yet hadn't.

I can't be the only person who gets on and off the scales if I'm not happy with what I see. Who only weighs on a Tuesday morning after I have had a wee and before I have a cup of tea? And has to have said scales on a certain place on the bathroom floor? We all have our quirky relationships with the scales. Be mindful that they don't sabotage your weight loss by making you feel low if they don't provide a lower number.

I have added a tracker at the end of the book should you wish to track your weight with some supportive things to think about.

Whatever you decide to do, make sure it suits you and supports your mindset and your weight loss.

Ker-ching,
Positive Polly
earns her
keep

X

22

SILVER COINS

Throughout our whole process of surgery and weight loss, we will have moments where we may be anxious or derailed for a moment, a day or two or longer. This is natural. This doesn't mean that something negative has caused this, it could be something really positive. However, because we are not sure how to deal with the new positive situation, we can either let it affect us negatively, or we can dismiss its positive energy, not utilising the situation to our full advantage.

What do I really mean by this? Let me give you an example.

Say you are three stone down in weight loss and you are having a day where you just can't see through your own eyes how wonderfully well you are doing. It may be that all you can see is the old you, or you are not quite sure how to dress now you are shrinking. It may be that all of your clothes are suddenly too big for you and you are feeling a bit meh! Then someone comes along and says *"Faye/Frank! Look at you. You are looking great. I can really see you have lost weight."* There are two reactions that could happen now to this comment.

I have a Positive Polly and a Negative Nelly who jostle for position within my mind. The Positive Polly would think *"Yes! Thank you! I am doing really well and I really appreciate your comments and for letting me know!"* She would accept their comment and would provide a nice comment in return.

The Negative Nelly would think *"Yeah sure, you are just saying that to be kind, or are you being sarcastic? Yes that's it, you are having a dig"* and dismiss the positive comment and change the subject.

I went through phases. Sometimes Positive Polly was in charge and sometimes Negative Nelly was in charge. To this day, little old Negative Nelly can still creep up on me from time to time, though I keep Negative Nelly more in check these days.

I learnt an incredible lesson from a beautiful friend about stacking up or collecting silver coins in your mind. This was a lady who I became friends with as we lived next door to each other and had children the same age. We went on to support each other through a variety of life's challenges and would spend wonderful times together with and without our children. She taught me many things as we approached life from different perspectives. Despite now living in a different country, she is still a wonderful friend and I still use the silver coin lesson I am about to share with you.

The Silver Coin lesson is: With each positive comment you receive, you hypothetically accept it as a silver coin. The more positive responses you give, to a positive or negative comment, the more silver coins you attract. So for all and any comments, my aim is to be positive in return and keep collecting and stacking my silver coins.

Do you think it sounds crazy? Try it. For everything and anything that anyone says to you that is positive, gracefully and positively accept that comment and think of that silver coin dropping onto your stack. For anything they say that is negative, especially about your weight, your surgery, your progress, or anything else, respond with a positive comment and ka-ching. Hear that silver penny drop into your collection.

Let's try it together. Let's pretend your name is Anna and you are having a chat with Courtney.

Courtney: *"Hey Anna, how are you?"*

Anna (you): *"I'm really well thank you, (coin 1) how are you and the kids?"*

Courtney: *"We are good, Tom had a cold but is better now. Hey, you are looking really well, (coin 2) are you losing weight?"*

Anna (you): *"Oh poor Tom, there's so much going around. (deep breath) Thank you, yes I am. I'm really enjoying feeling more me (coin 3). Your hair is looking nice (Ka-Ching! Your 4th coin drops into your pile)"*

Courtney: *"That's great. Oh, thank you (coin 5), I go to Mark on Smith Street, he is great you know"*

Anna (you): *"Oh nice I will have to take a look one day, see you soon."*

The more you train your mind to respond positively about the new you, the more positive currency you will have in your bank to deal with any negative comments. Ready to practise?

Courtney: *"Hey Anna, how are you?"*

Anna (you): *"I'm really well thank you (coin 1), how are you and the kids?"*

Courtney: *"We are good, Tom had a cold but is better now. Hey, you are looking slimmer, get you, are you losing weight? You had got quite, well, you know, big, after you changed jobs"*

Anna (you): *"Oh poor Tom, there's so much going around. (deep breath) Thank you (coin 2), yes, I am doing well (coin 3) (Emma now does not need to know any more of your information, you just now hit them with a Positive Polly comment). Your hair is looking nice (Ka-Ching! Coin 4 drops into your pile)"*

Courtney: *"Oh, oh erm, thank you (coin 5), I go to Mark on Smith Street, he is great you know"*

Anna (you): *"Oh nice. I will have to take a look one day, see you soon"*

And that, my friends, is the best way to deal with the Negative Nellys of the world along with the Courtneys, who could be a family member (we all have them) or a "friend" or even some random person at the supermarket.

Collect those silver coins. Make yourself positively rich.

*Note I don't actually know anyone called Anna or Courtney.

Keep your eyes
on the prize,
and
ALWAYS
move forward

X

ONWARDS

As we come to the end of our time together in this book, I want to personally say, directly to each of you, that no matter what stage you are at on your journey with gastric surgery, with the right research and consideration at each stage of the journey, you will make the best choices for yourself. Even if that is to not have gastric surgery.

Gastric surgery is a journey. It isn't a cop-out and it certainly isn't a quick fix. Remember that it is an effective tool, to enable you to lose weight. Your gastric surgery provides you with the internal tool to manage that weight loss for a sustained, lighter future.

Should you need to, you can refer to this book time and time again. Make notes in the margins, and fold the corners of the pages to remind you where to re-read. I have created a fabulous workbook with journal sections for each chapter which is available through www.gastricsurgery-thelivedexperience.com and refine your lifestyle to suit you and your body.

Stay in touch with me as you document your own journey. Tag me so I can be your cheerleader at Gastric Surgery: The Lived Experience on Facebook and Instagram and come along and join us on our beautiful website. See 'Connect With Me' over the page.

There will be multiple gastric and bariatric forums out there that if you ask the right questions will give you sound answers. However, using my lived experience, I have hopefully covered all of the basics and more to support you through **your** lived experience.

An amazing person supported me through a tricky period of time. She was calm, understanding, clear, honest and relatable. She delivered her thoughts and guidance in the correct fashion, from a place of integrity and had a saying at the end of every period of time that I had with her which was, **"onwards"**.

Continue to invest in yourself through all of the ways mentioned and through the Gastric Surgery: The Lived Experience, Success Sessions, Workshops and Membership you will have everything at your fingertips to support your ongoing success.

So to you, my friend, my fellow gastric surgery member, **onwards**, to your own successful Gastric Surgery Lived Experience. To a successful lighter and brighter new you.

I really hope you gain as much
from reading this book
as I have from sharing
my journey with you.

Whichever direction
your gastric surgery journey takes you,
I wish you ALL the love
for the most success

Louise

x

The most successful
futures are
with those
who are
in the same tribe

X

CONNECT WITH ME

https://gastricsurgerythelivedexperience.com

Facebook: Gastric Surgery: The Lived Experience

Instagram: GastricSurgery_livedexperience

https://www.youtube.com/@
gastricsurgery_livedexperience

Invest in yourself
as much
as you would
invest in
others you love

X

Louise Neil is a gastric surgery patient, a qualified educator, success coach and entrepreneur. She is happily married with two children.

Louise wasn't always in this position though. The year Louise had her gastric surgery, her marriage had failed and it was only a matter of time before she decided she was ready and strong enough to step away and make a life for herself and her children. She was working part-time, desperately juggling work and parenting, whilst studying to become a qualified educator so that she could progress her career.

Louise had suffered for many years with her weight and from the moment Louise decided to have surgery, she also decided that there would be more to life from then on. Through sheer determination, she has become the successful woman she is today, with a great career and happily remarried to a lovely man.

As Louise prepared herself for her new life pre and post-surgery, she realised that there were no first-hand stories out there, by people who had lived the experience, to help her understand the process a little better. Her mind was made up, she would ensure she would support others through their gastric surgery journey for many years to come.

Today, Louise works with people all over the world to ensure they achieve their own goals with their gastric surgery, helping them through obstacles that hinder their dreams of successful and sustained weight loss, so that they can free themselves from the ties of the past, allowing them to live the life they want to live, which often ties in with their progress beyond gastric surgery. Louise's coaching far extends that of gastric surgery success.

Find Louise at www.gastricsurgerythelivedexperience.com and benefit from her lived experience, coaching and success membership.

Yum, yum,
bubble gum,
nourishing foods
in my tum

x

MY USUAL DAY OF FOOD AND DRINK

This does depend on what I have booked in my diary for the day, so I will give you some examples of the foods I choose from, it can change with the seasons and with what I fancy:

BREAKFAST CHOICES

2 x eggs either, scrambled, boiled or poached with 1 x crispbread spread with butter;

250ml milk mixed with a shake powder which is a nutritionally based powder with added protein;

Avocado, eggs and fish. Any fish depending on what I have available;

1 x egg with mushrooms;

Omelette, either hot or cold;

Latte and a protein bar or balls

Porridge

Fruit and natural yoghurt with seeds and nuts

Garlic and herb cream cheese on crispbreads with smoked salmon and spinach leaves (I love this and my hubby invented it for me).

LUNCH & DINNERS

Any selection from breakfast;

Baked Beans and crispbread or half a slice of toast (max);

Protein pasta with any sauce;

Jacket potato with tuna and mayo or baked beans;

Lentil and mixed bean Chilli Con Carne;

Soups - I either make them in my soup maker (best kitchen utensil ever) or buy them and look for high protein;

Meat/fish/poultry with vegetables and a cheese sauce;

Steak

Roast dinner;

Spaghetti Bolognese with protein pasta;

Shepards Pie loaded with lentils;

Salads - Cottage cheese, fish, chicken or any leftover meats;

Pasta with prawns and a tomato and pesto sauce.

Traybakes like aubergine, lentils and tomato sauce.

SNACKS I ENJOY

Raspberries;

Blueberries;

Yoghurts;

BabyBel;

Cheese spread or hard cheese on crispbreads;

Hummus and thinly sliced cucumber;

Milk - warm or cold;

A high-protein, low sugar, shake made with milk;

Protein nut bars.

DRINKS ACROSS THE DAY

Water;

Collagen drink;

Tea;

Coffee;

Sugar-free drinks;

Milk;

Alcohol on occasion (not across every day, haha).

From the above, we make all sorts of meals, as a couple and for the family. I simply have a smaller amount and I always prioritise protein and vitamins from veg, salad and fruit. Carbohydrates come last.

Please do not feel that you have to use this tracker. Only track your weight if it will be of benefit to you. You may want to make a note of your inches too.

SUCCESS TRACKER

Starting Date
Starting weight
End of LRD weight

Date	Current Weight	Total of Lbs /Kgs lost	How are you feeling?	What will you improve for next week's success?

Date	Current Weight	Total of Lbs /Kgs lost	How are you feeling?	What will you improve for next week's success?

Your success is down
to you and your
commitment to

YOURSELF

x

I am with you

every step

of the way

x

Printed in Great Britain
by Amazon